A Beginner's Guide to the Magic of Herbal Medicine

Kynleex O. Allen

The origins and advantages of herbal medicine

An essential and significant component of alternative medicine is herbal medicine. It is an integral component of alternative therapeutic approaches. A variety of plant parts are used in herbal medicine. plant components with medicinal qualities.

The leaves, stem, fruits, seeds, flowers, and roots are a few of these components.

The chemical compounds that give plants their medicinal properties are present in plants naturally.

When these chemicals are introduced into the body, these nutrients fill in any nutritional deficiencies. Herbal medicine has both curative and preventive effects.

In a way, herbs are similar to the vegetables we eat every day. Food would indeed have turned into medicine if we consumed them with the knowledge and purpose of preventing disease(s).

One of the oldest types of medicine in existence is herbal medicine. In fact, it has received extensive research and documentation in some international locations.

For instance, Ayurvedic medicine is practiced in India and Chinese Traditional Herbal Medicine is practiced in China. It is also widely utilized in other Asian and European nations.

In Africa, which is closer to home, various African nations have long used a variety of herbs for the treatment of various diseases.

The lack of thorough documentation is the main issue with herbal medicine in Nigeria. Practitioners across the nation have passed away without preserving their knowledge of herbal medicine for future generations.

I have no doubt that this trend is about to change because I observe a lot of it being produced by modern practitioners.

For centuries, people have used herbal medicine to treat a wide range of illnesses.

Nature has endowed humans with an enormous variety of herbs, all of which are loaded with medicinal benefits that can be used for the treatment and prevention of a wide range of illnesses.

To put it mildly, the rate at which herbal medicine has become more and more popular is alarming. It's also crucial to remember that the current popularity of herbal medicine is supported by hard data and firsthand accounts.

This only serves to support the findings that scientists like Dr. Batmangheldj had consistently made known during his lifetime. He claimed that because the human body is a part of nature, only natural substances—not inorganic chemical drugs—can heal it.

Benefits of herbal medicine include:

Herbal products are more affordable and cost-effective than pharmaceuticals, which are becoming so expensive that the average person can hardly afford them.

Herbal medicine is now a viable alternative to modern medicine due to the growing body of evidence supporting its growing effectiveness and much lower incidence of side effects.

It is simple to find herbal products in the form of supplements, herbal teas, extracts, essential oils, and so on. They can be found online, at pharmacy stores, in health food stores that are opening up all over the place.

Additionally, since they are plant-based products, you do not need a prescription to purchase them. Additionally, in America, supplements are not required to be registered with the FDA or to undergo testing prior to use.

Whatever the case, it is our responsibility as consumers to make sure we buy our products from reputable stores. Additionally, the goods must be produced and packaged by reputable businesses. Always make sure you thoroughly read the labels on the supplements' bottles and packets.

These herbs have been found to be effective in treating a number of diseases. Their effectiveness has been supported by a number of studies.

There are herbs that can be used to treat both simple ailments like the common cold and more severe ones like cancer, diabetes, and cardiovascular diseases.

Immune system stimulation: Herbal products don't obstruct the body's natural physiological functions. Instead, they encourage such procedures.

Particularly, herbal products strengthen the immune system due to their chemical constituents. They collaborate with every component of the system to improve its performance. By providing enough antioxidants, they, for instance, support the antioxidant immune system.

Do you constantly have the flu? You may benefit from using herbal medicine. Goldenseal and echinacea both have anti-infective properties that support the immune system. To treat the flu and the common cold, we advise using this herb.

A woman's life will inevitably include the incredibly frustrating experience of menopause. Hot flashes, cold sweats, weight gain, and insomnia are just a few of the symptoms brought on by the abrupt change in estrogen levels.

We use the North American herbal remedy black cohosh to help you get relief from menopause symptoms.

Although it's simple to overlook, good blood circulation is crucial for your health and wellbeing. It speaks to the effectiveness with which blood and oxygen circulate through the body.

Your muscles, tissues, and organs receive the hormones and nutrients they require from circulation. It is essential for your body's capacity to eliminate cellular waste.

The adaptable herb ginkgo biloba increases circulation and aids the body's defense against inflammation.

Ginkgo biloba and comparable herbs also promote brain health. Thus, using herbal remedies may help you remember things better and pay attention for longer.

Any medical expert will tell you that stress management is crucial for virtually every aspect of your health. Happily, stress relief is closer than you might realize. One of the most well-liked medicinal herb varieties, ginseng, has excelled as a stress-relieving treatment.

Do you get tired of having to rely on the coffee maker to get you through the day? Traditional energy boosters only provide short-term bursts of energy, and some of them can be harmful to your health.

On the other hand, herbal medicine offers you potent energy-boosting components that give you a consistent source of energy without requiring you to give up your other health and wellness objectives. We usually suggest ginseng if you suffer from persistent fatigue.

Contents

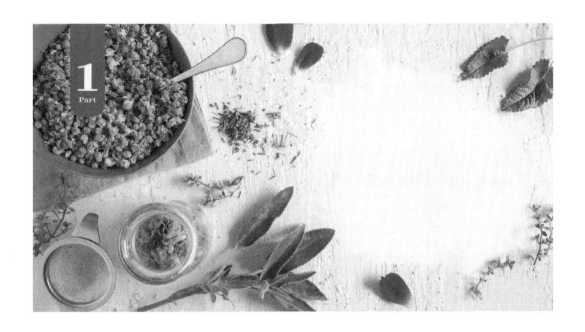

Part 1

Herbal Medicine in Four Steps

Herbalism isn't rocket science, but it *is* science. Our ancestors knew a lot more about health and the human body than popular culture gives them credit for, and the practice of herbalism is the collected wisdom of centuries of trial and error. There are still some aspects of herbalism we haven't yet explained with science, but it's not "magic." Herbalists work with plants because the vitamins, minerals, and organic chemicals that plants create to keep themselves healthy can keep humans healthy, too.

Because herbs are so complex, it's not accurate to think of them as "weak" or "gentle" drugs. They fit into a complete system of health care that is not the same as the mainstream Western model. The holistic herbal model prioritizes early preventive care, and when illness happens, it focuses on supporting and strengthening the body's own response mechanisms.

Just because herbalism is a different system doesn't mean you have to choose one or the other. Think of it like fusion cuisine—taking the tastiest parts of one type of food and blending them with another to get an exciting, delicious new style. Most strategies we include here can be complementary to other treatments you're receiving.

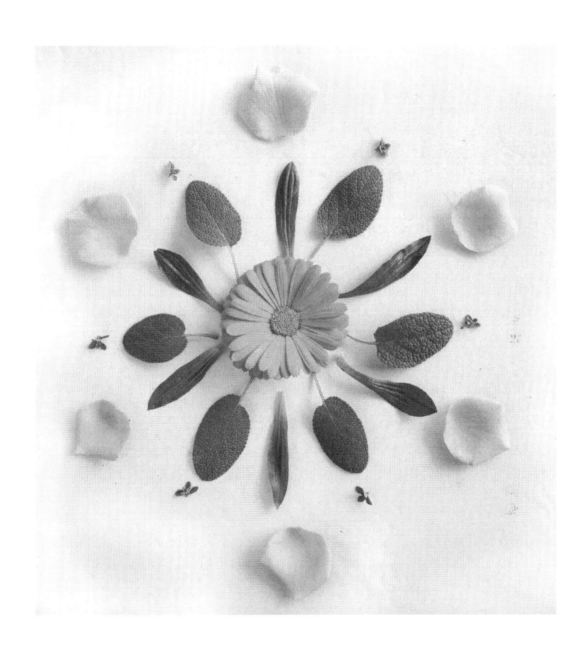

STEP ONE
Learn What You Need

Herbs are suited to different bodies and different purposes, but they're all multitalented. If you find yourself working with an herb that doesn't taste good to you, it's okay. You can choose another herb and see if that suits your taste better. Because herbs have so many gifts, it's usually possible to find one that you'll find helpful and enjoyable. Exploring herbal medicine can be fun, so go with what feels good to you. Over time, you'll learn what suits your needs best. In the meantime, enjoy the ride!

The Best Herbs for Your Body

There are many ways to define the "best" herb for your body, but it always comes down to one very practical guideline: "The best herb is the one you'll actually take!"

A Holistic Approach to Healing

You can make herbal tea out of just one herb and get all the benefits of that one herb. Or, you can blend several herbs into a formula for a synergistic effect that is greater than any one of those herbs on its own.

The same is true of health. You could take an herbal approach, adding an herbal tea or tincture blend to your daily routine. And you can expand that to a holistic approach—you might add more unprocessed whole foods to your diet, find time each day to go for a walk or meditate, and make an effort to get an extra hour of sleep each night. Sure, simply adding herbs into your daily routine is a great step toward a healthier you, and sometimes, in this busy life, it's all there is time for. But those herbs can be even more effective when they're part of a whole "formula" of healthy habits.

In our school and clinic, we consider four areas when trying to help people build their health: **sleep**, **food**, **stress**, and **movement**. Why these four? Because in our modern lifestyles, these are areas that usually need some support: Our lives are busy and stressful, which means most people don't get as much sleep as they need and don't have the time for wholesome, home-cooked meals every day. As many people work in offices, there isn't always the chance to get enough movement throughout the day, and, with all that's going on, it can be difficult to manage stress well. We find that when we can make any positive change in any of these areas, it greatly enhances the work we're doing with herbs.

We don't necessarily do it all at once—that can be overwhelming. Instead, we like to place each area on a compass and just keep going around the circle: Is there anything we can improve here, either by adding herbs or with lifestyle changes—or both? If so, great, and if not, we move on to the next. Not everything has to be perfect, but the more we can move in a positive direction, the more momentum we build and the stronger we get. Herbs can be the first step in that direction or part of a holistic protocol for a healthier life!

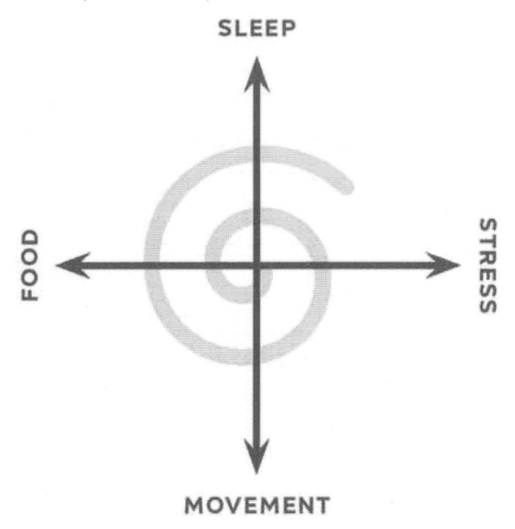

How Herbal Energetics Affect Their Applications

The fundamental basis of the system of herbal medicine is *energetics*—an old word that basically means "how we categorize what herbs do, and what your body needs." Long before we invented laboratory testing, we needed a system to determine what was ailing the body and what actions should be taken to address it. Over time, people learned to categorize symptoms and illnesses based on things that could be determined with the senses: hot or cold, damp or dry, tense or lax. Our five senses were our original scientific tools! Although it's simple, this system still holds up today.

We can talk about inflammation, for example, as heat: Imagine you've been stung by a bee, and you have a red welt where the sting was. That welt is warm to the touch. There's a benefit to that warmth —blood rushing to the area will carry away the bee's venom, and, assuming you're not allergic, the issue is resolved reasonably quickly. But that flood of warmth—*that inflammation*—is problematic if it runs out of control. In that case, it needs to be cooled down, so we would look for herbs with cooling effects, such as rose. And you may have done just that without herbs: Ice on a bee sting is very soothing! No one had to teach you to put ice on it; it was intuitive. Your senses told you that ice would cool down that hot, irritated sting.

ENERGETICS

HOT Inflamed, irritated tissue, including fever and burns. Anything that literally feels hot, agitated, or overly fast (such as palpitations or racing thoughts).

COLD Slowness of function, whether that's circulation, digestion, or thought. This includes depression, hypothyroidism, and anything that literally feels cold.

DAMP Too much fluid anywhere in the body, such as a swollen sprained ankle, edema, rheumatism in the joints, and bloating.

DRY Not enough fluid anywhere in the body, including dry mouth, "frayed" nerves, and all types of dry skin.

TENSE Too much tightness anywhere in the body, including muscle tension, pinched nerves, and tension headaches.

LAX Not enough tension anywhere in the body, including any kind of prolapse, diarrhea, and even wrinkled aging skin.

For another example, let's say you've sprained your ankle. There's inflammation, which is heat—you see the redness and you feel the warmth of the blood rushing in. But there's more: There's also lymphatic fluid rushing to carry away the damaged cells so new cells can be built. All that extra fluid makes your sprained ankle puffy and swollen—it's damp. You can feel the extra fluid inside, and that extra fluid becomes uncomfortable—you want it to drain away. You might elevate your foot to help that drainage, which is a great idea. You can also work with drying, or astringent, herbs to help "squeeze out" the fluids through the lymphatic system.

We can identify health issues by these aspects—a fever is hot, or a headache might be a result of tension. We can also put herbs into these same categories by their effects—ginger and cayenne are warming herbs, for example. There's a third aspect here, called "constitution," meaning "your normal state." Maybe you're a person who is always warm—for example, you consistently feel comfortable in a T-shirt in winter. We can say you have a "hot" constitution. Or you might be the opposite—the first person to put on a sweater, and always dressed in layers. We can say you have a "cold" constitution. Your constitution might have more than one aspect: You might run cold, and you might also have slow circulation, which makes you prone to edema or varicose veins in your legs. We can say you are "cold and damp." No one constitution is ideal, or better, than any other—it's just your body. The key is to keep it from swinging too far out of balance.

Knowing your constitution is quite handy. Let's say you're a person with a strong tendency toward dryness—a dry constitution. When you read about all the great ways nettle can help and nourish, you might be very excited to try it. But nettle is drying, and if you drink a lot of it, you might find your natural dryness is exaggerated, which can be uncomfortable. That doesn't mean you can't have nettle tea—it just means that when you work with drying herbs over the long term, you'll need to add a moistening herb, such as linden or marshmallow, to balance the dryness.

Not sure? Don't worry, your body will tell you! If you start drinking nettle tea every day and you have a damp constitution, nettle's dryness will help drain some of your dampness, which will probably feel good. If you have a dry constitution, you might see benefits from the nourishment of nettles but also feel extra dry. Your body is telling you what to do—just add a moistening herb and continue on your way! The herbs we include in this book are very forgiving, so feel free to experiment, and if you need to make an adjustment along the way, you can.

Choosing the Best Herbs for Your Needs

Based on this energetic information, you can choose the best herb for your situation, even if you don't know the medical diagnostic name for what's going on. You may not know why, for example, you have a runny nose, but you do know that it's damp and lax (flowing), so you might consider a drying, astringent herb to help dry and tighten the mucous membranes.

At first, thinking this way about health may seem a little awkward —it's not how most of us were raised to think about our bodies. But learning to identify health issues this way gives you the independence to start applying the herbs you learn about even to things that aren't in this book. To help you with that, we define each ailment with its energetic terms, so, as you study each one, you'll start to see how they fit into the herbal energetic system.

We've done the same for each herb, too. Many herbs are quite obvious, such as ginger—definitely hot. But some herbs are more subtle, and it takes a while to learn exactly how to categorize them. That categorization can usually be felt on your tongue—just like you can taste the astringency of an unripe banana—so the more you practice, the better you'll get at it!

Single Herbs versus Herbal Blends

It's always okay to work with one herb at a time, but sometimes you want to blend herbs together. For example, there may be more than one herb helpful for your situation, and you may want to try them together. Or you may want to balance an herb that is very warming or drying with herbs that are somewhat cooling or moistening to align with your constitution.

Working with herbs is very much like cooking, and you won't know if you like it until you try it. If you like your recipes very precise, use the formulas in part 3. If you prefer to just "eyeball it" when you cook, use that same approach to herbal formulation, keeping the basic energetic principles in mind.

As you go through the book, you might be inclined to think that every herb is exactly the herb you need—right now! Don't worry, this feeling is normal and happens to us, too: It's just so exciting to see so many helpful plants that we want to try them all. But it's a good idea to keep your immediate goal in mind, and focus on it. Start with a target of three to five herbs in any formula—for example, if you want to make a formula for anxiety, even though there are a lot of great herbs that can help, pick the three that seem most applicable to your situation, and start with those. Just like cooking and baking, start with a small batch to make sure you like it. If you do, make a larger batch and enjoy it over time. You might like to keep a "recipe book" of all your herbal experiments, so you can recreate the ones you like best whenever you want.

And if all that feels too difficult, just stick to one herb at a time. It's still a very effective way to work with herbs, and it allows you to get to know each herb in depth.

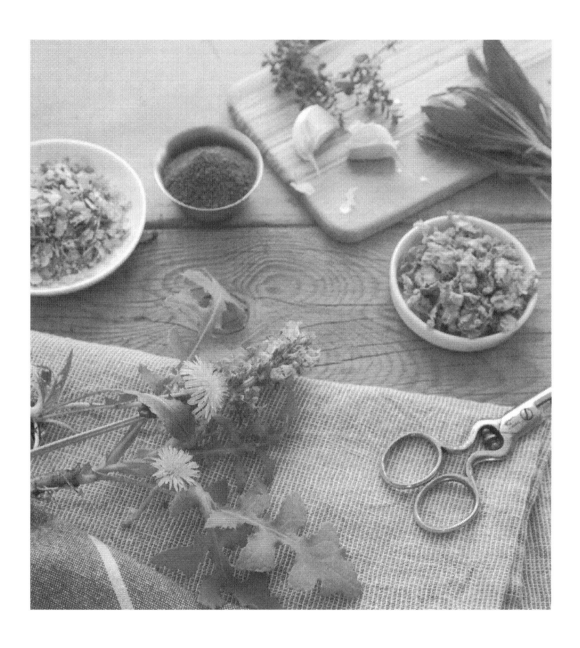

STEP TWO
Source Your Medicinal Herbs

The quality of your herbs matters! When you shop
for fruits and vegetables, you are careful to choose
the ones that have vibrant colors and no bruising
or "bad spots." The same applies to your herb
selection: Always look for vibrant colors, aromas,
and flavor from your herbs.

Common Forms of Medicinal Herbs

Herbs come in several forms. You can purchase dried herbs whole or in "cut and sifted" form, which basically means the dried plants are chopped up like confetti. This is a great way to blend herbs for tea or to make tinctures. You can purchase herbs fresh from local farms or even grow them in your garden, which is great if you're planning to make tinctures or oils. Fresh herbs can also be made into tea and, of course, added to food. You may already be familiar with powdered herbs from the spice section of the grocery store: They're in small containers because once an herb is powdered, it loses its potency more quickly. And, of course, some herbs are sold as food, such as candied ginger, cayenne peppers, garlic, etc.

The Herbalist's Philosophy

We like to avoid the word "use" in reference to herbs whenever possible. To "use" something implies exploitation. We view herbs as teachers, allies, and friends, not mere resources to be exploited. We don't *use* our human friends to help us move or plan a party—we work together with them. We feel the same way about plants, and try to reflect that in the way we speak and write about them.

This is one small aspect of an ongoing effort to respect plants as living, independent organisms with their own needs and desires. While plants don't perceive or act on the world the same way we do, they are nevertheless alive and responsive to their environments. (The books *What a Plant Knows*, by Daniel Chamovitz, and *The Hidden Life of Trees*, by Peter Wohlleben, are excellent explorations of plant sense and sensitivity.) It's our responsibility as stewards and caretakers to make sure we take only what we need, minimize waste, and actively restore plant habitats and populations so these beings can continue to share their gifts with us for generations to come.

Shopping for Your Herbs

High-quality herbs are high-quality herbs, regardless of their source. Where you live, that might be a local health food store, a small local farm, or even your neighbor's garden. You may even have an herb shop in your town. You might be surprised to find that your grocery store has good-quality herbs, too, especially those frequently sold as produce. Or you may live somewhere with limited access to herbs, in which case you'll find reputable online retailers in the <u>Resources</u> section.

You'll also find that the price of herbs can vary greatly, depending on where you purchase them. Cheaper is not usually better! Local small producers often have to charge more for their herbs and herbal products, but the quality is also often much higher.

Experiment with small batches first, so you learn which producers have the best quality; that will help you know whether it's worth the money.

ETHICAL SOURCING AND PROTECTING AT-RISK PLANTS

Some herbs should be avoided altogether, because they are at risk of extinction from overharvesting and habitat destruction. Many plants, especially woodland plants, require healthy forests to grow in and can't be cultivated. Some of these plants, such as goldenseal, osha, and black or blue cohosh, are very popular and are still being sold. However, just like vegetables, there are many herbs with similar qualities, so there's no need to purchase these at-risk plants. You can learn more about at-risk herbs and those that should be avoided at the United Plant Savers website, <u>unitedplantsavers.org</u>.

Some popular herbs should also be avoided because their sale exploits the people and communities they come from. In general, when there's a new trendy "superfood" from some far-off place, we avoid it. Maca is an example: Touted as a plant that will give you more energy, and that is also quite delicious, people flocked to it. But maca is a subsistence food for the indigenous Peruvians living at high altitudes, and the more that industrialized nations purchase, the more expensive it becomes: Local people can no longer afford to eat it. Issues like this are complicated, but when it comes to exotic superfoods, it's always good to remember we have our own superfoods right here. Plants such as cranberries, nettle, and dandelion leaves don't have the exotic appeal, but they're every bit as super!

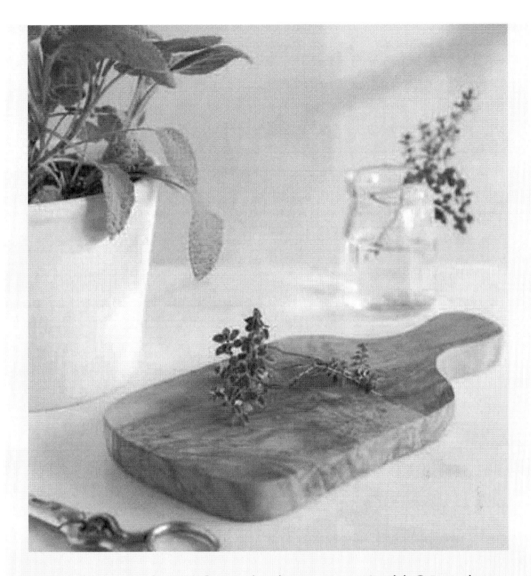

How can you know if your herbs are sustainable? Buy them as locally as possible, and know your farmer. If there's an exotic herb you're interested in, research it and find fair-trade sources. And always be on the lookout for local herbs that can do the same work! In this way, we can do our part to make sure herbalism remains a sustainable and healthy practice, not just for our own bodies, but for the body of the whole earth as well.

What to Avoid

There are a few things to keep in mind when sourcing herbs: soil quality, growing practices, and how the herbs are dried or processed.

If the soil where the herbs are grown is contaminated with heavy metals or other pollution, this is likely to be in the plant matter. It's important to know where the herbs were grown, so you can determine whether the soil was clean. This can be a problem for herbs grown anywhere, but especially those grown in places that don't have regulations about soil pollution. Some larger herb retailers, such as Mountain Rose Herbs, test their herbs to make sure they are free of soil-based contamination.

You might be disinclined to purchase herbs grown in urban farms, but don't write them off: Talk to the producers and ask about their soil. Most urban farms bring in clean soil and use water filtration to make sure their produce is safe.

Growing practices are also important. How were insects managed? What kind of fertilizer was used? Were the herbs grown in a greenhouse or outdoors? Were they grown hydroponically or in soil? All these things have pros and cons, but the bottom line is the result: If the herbs have vibrant color and strong aromas and flavors, then the quality is good.

The drying and processing step can be tricky, too: High-quality herbs can be ruined if they're dried at too high a temperature or stored improperly. You'll know this is the case if there is significant browning in the dried herbs. This is the same browning you would see on a living plant that had a brown, dried leaf—it looks un-vital. Let's use St. John's wort as an example: This plant should have some brown when it's dried, but its brown color is a deep-red mahogany. That's very different from the brown-black color of basil leaves that have gone bad in your refrigerator. The latter is the one to avoid.

The bottom line is, know who you're buying your herbs from. Ask about their growing practices, about the soil and water, and about their processing practices. Not only does this help you make good choices, but it also helps build community between the people who grow our herbs (and food) and those of us who consume them. When we understand more about where our herbs come from, we value them, our farmers, and our environment more.

Ideas for Growing, Wildcrafting, and Harvesting Herbs

It's always okay to purchase (vs. grow) your herbs, and in today's busy lifestyle that's often the easiest way to get herbs into your life. But it's also lovely to develop a relationship with the herbs you love while they're still alive—whether you grow them in your garden or find them in the wild. Even if you don't harvest them at all, getting to know your herbs as living plants brings a new dimension to your practice of herbalism.

Herb Garden

No matter how urban your surroundings, you can grow your own herbs. There are many herbs that will grow happily in a pot near a sunny window—you don't even need a yard! If you've never grown any kind of plant before, or if you've ever described yourself as having a "brown thumb," don't worry: Growing plants is just like any other thing you want to do. Spend a little time on it each day, and soon enough it will seem easy.

Some herbs are definitely easier to grow than others. Mint, catnip, sage, and yarrow are easy ones to start with and can be found as seedlings or seeds at your local garden center. Mint and catnip are very easy to grow indoors as well. All are perfectly happy to live in pots if you don't have a yard or if you don't have safe soil to grow in. You can have your soil tested with your local Extension Office—they'll send you a testing kit and provide results about soil safety as well as tips about the best type of fertilizer to use with the type of soil you have—all for about $10. Your local Extension Office also offers classes and advice about gardening in your area, as well as many other services, for free or at a low cost. (You can search "county extension office" to find the one near you.)

Even though it's not an herb, pothos is a good plant to practice with. You can find it at your local garden center, or even in many grocery stores. It's a simple green leaf, sometimes with white markings, that has a habit of forming vines and is very pretty. More importantly, though, pothos is a good practice plant because it can live in nearly any circumstances—dark rooms or sunny windows—and it tolerates under- and overwatering. Not only that, but it improves indoor air quality. If you've never grown anything before, pothos can help you build confidence to grow your own herbs.

Just like with herbalism, the best way to get started growing herbs is just to start! Buy a seedling, put it in a pot with some good dirt and a little water, and check on it every day. Plants are living beings, and you'll learn to "hear" your plant's communication in the same way you learn to understand what your cat or dog is trying to tell you!

Wildcrafting

Although it's alluring to think about hiking out into wild places and harvesting your own herbs, most times, the best advice we can give is, actually, not to do this.

There are some very abundant and fairly safe herbs to wildcraft, but overharvesting is a serious problem for our wild herbs, and when so many can be organically cultivated, it is really much better to do that instead of taking plants from the wild.

When we dry aerial parts, we put them mostly whole into brown paper bags. Once they're completely dry, we use scissors to cut them up while they're still in the bags. This way, bits of plant don't end up all over the kitchen.

We live in a very humid region. If we have some plants drying and the weather turns rainy, we put the brown bags on a laundry drying rack, with a small space heater underneath to keep them from absorbing all the moisture in the air.

However, it is very rewarding to find wild plants and work with them, so here are some guidelines for doing so safely—for you, for the plants, and for the ecosystem they are a part of!

Identify the plant. Before anything else, it's important to know what you've found. Learning to identify plants accurately takes time, but, if you practice, you will be able to do it just as easily as you recognize your friend across a crowded room! There are some excellent books on plant identification in the Resources section. We also recommend attending local plant walks. These walks, usually offered by local herbalists, typically include looking at the plants where they grow and learning how to identify and work with each plant. They are a great way to test your plant ID skills.

Get permission to harvest. If you find some plants you want to harvest, obtain permission from the property owners. Depending on where you live, wild land may be public or private—either way, there may be people there who harvest herbs already. If the land is private, ask the owners, and if the land is public, try to find out if anyone is already harvesting there, including wild animals. And, of course, make sure the location is protected from environmental hazards—for example, along the side of a road is not a good place to harvest plants, although you will find many growing there!

Harvest responsibly. Herbs are more than just medicine for humans: They are part of the complex, interconnected, living world we share. Sometimes those plants are healing the ecosystem they live in, and their medicine is not for us. The plants we call herbs are also often food and medicine for many species of animals in the area, from the smallest pollinator to the largest mammal.

Twenty years ago, herbalists used to teach: one-third for the herbalist, one-third for the animals, and one-third for seed—but that rule does not work well for wild harvesting anymore. First, there are a lot more herbalists today, and if every herbalist takes one-third, eventually there will be none left. Also, many plant species struggle in our current climate, so they are just not as abundant as they once were. Animals struggle, too, and depend on the plants to survive. Today, better guidelines might be: If this plant literally grows as far as you can see, it is safe to take a small amount, and harvest in such a way that it looks like you were not there. These guidelines help us be more aware of our impact.

Be aware of a particular area over time. Perhaps you find what seems like a lot of a certain plant, but because you may not have seen it in previous years, you don't realize it is in decline. Plants have years of abundance and years of difficulty, just like people. It is a good idea to visit an area where you'd like to harvest over several years to get a feel for the health of those plants and their ecosystem over time. If it's a tough year, there may not be enough of that plant to sustain the animals who depend on it and to allow the plant to reseed for next year if we herbalists also harvest some. The time you spend building this relationship with the ecosystem is well spent: You will learn far more than just what kind of year the plants are having. This kind of relationship to place used to be an integral part of being human—rebuilding it can be extremely nourishing and medicinal, even if you never harvest a single plant!

Harvesting

When you harvest plants, whether grown yourself or found in a sustainable wild place, it's important to process them appropriately so you don't waste the plants. If you're harvesting roots, wash them well and cut them immediately: Roots can become very difficult, or even nearly impossible, to cut once they've dried. You can make a tincture or oil with them immediately, or dry them for tea or tincturing later. Dry them in a dehydrator if you have one. If not, dry them in a brown paper bag put in a warm, dry place, and check often for mold. If mold develops, remove the moldy pieces and find a drier location.

If harvesting aerial parts (leaves, stems, flowers—anything that grows aboveground), you can make an oil or tincture with them immediately, dry them for tea or tincturing later, or just eat them as food. Unless they are visibly dirty, we don't typically wash aerial parts: Adding water just makes them more difficult to dry and more likely to mold. Dry them in a dehydrator, if you have one, or in a brown paper bag put in a warm, dry place, such as an attic. If you live in a humid region, be very attentive for mold.

Make sure your herbs are thoroughly dried before storing them in airtight glass containers.

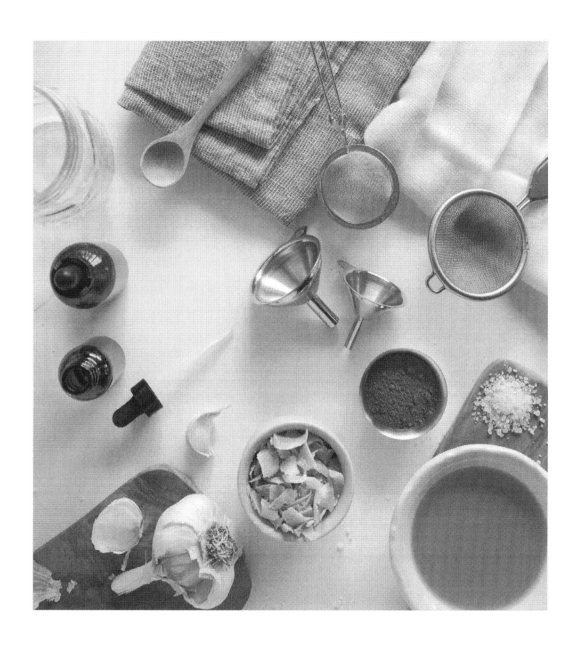

STEP THREE
Make Your Herbal Medicine

Making herbal medicines is easy and fun. With a few simple tools and ingredients, you can transform your herbs into all manner of delicious and effective remedies.

Tools, Equipment, and Ingredients

It doesn't take fancy equipment or rare, expensive ingredients to make high-quality herbal preparations. Most of what you'll need is probably already in your kitchen.

Essential Tools and Equipment

Mason jars. These are the herbalist's best friend. Because they're made of heat-resistant glass, you can pour boiling water right into them to make tea. They're also handy for making tinctures, storing herbs, and more. Quart- and pint-size jars are the most versatile, though for storing dry herbs you may want larger jars. Many store-bought foods (sauerkraut, salsa, etc.) come in mason jars—just hand wash or run them through the dishwasher and dry to reuse them.

Wire mesh strainers. For straining tea or pressing out tinctures, you'll want strainers of various sizes. Start with a few single-mug strainers for making one cup of tea at a time, as well as a larger, bowl-size strainer for filtering larger amounts of herb-infused liquids.

Cheesecloth. This is handy not only for straining and squeezing herbs you've infused into liquid but also for wrapping the herbs in a poultice.

Measuring cups and spoons. Cup, tablespoon, and teaspoon measures are all helpful, as well as some graduated measuring cups with pour spouts, which allow you to measure down to a quarter ounce.

Funnels. A set of small funnels is extremely helpful for getting tinctures and other liquids into bottles with small openings.

Bottles. For storing tinctures long term, amber or blue glass bottles are best. The "Boston round" type is a favorite for tinctures and other liquid remedies, but any shape will do. Get in the habit of

saving and reusing any colored glass bottles you come across—
there are a number of kombucha brands that come in amber glass,
for instance.

One- and two-fluid-ounce bottles are most convenient for dose
bottles, while storage bottles are usually 4 to 12 fluid ounces. For
storage, use plain bottle caps, but you'll need dropper tops for dose
bottles.

Labels. Label your remedies as soon as you make them. Address
labels are sufficient for most purposes—even a bit of masking tape
will do in a pinch.

Blender. For mixing lotions, breaking down bulky fresh plant matter,
and other purposes, a standard kitchen blender will serve just fine.

Nice-to-Have Equipment

These tools make it easier to integrate herbs into your life, especially
if you have a busy schedule, but they're not as necessary as those
preceding.

French press. This is our favorite tool for making herbal infusions. It
allows the herb material to float freely in the water and exposes a lot
of surface area for extraction (you just press down to easily
dispense filtered tea), and it is simple to clean.

Thermos. When traveling or bringing your tea to work, a good
thermos is an asset. There are versions that include a filter built
directly into the lid, so you can put the herbs and water directly into
the thermos together from the start.

Press pot. This is an insulated pot with a lever you press to dispense.
People usually put coffee or strained tea into these, though we've
found you can usually get away with putting herbs directly into the
pot, pouring in boiling water, and letting it infuse in there. It'll stay hot
all day, and you just dispense it by the cup. (Hold a little mesh

strainer under the spout to catch any herb bits that pass through the tube.)

Herb grinder. A simple, small coffee grinder served us well for many years, but if you plan to make a lot of herb powders you may want a larger, dedicated machine.

Helpful Ingredients

Herbs and water alone will serve for a great many remedies, but some preparations require additional ingredients.

Alcohol. Tinctures are mixtures of herb extracts and alcohol. We usually use vodka or brandy.

Apple cider vinegar. Always use this, rather than distilled white vinegar, for herb-infused vinegars, oxymels (a blend of vinegar and honey), and topical applications.

Honey. Choose local honey whenever possible, unprocessed/unfiltered if you can get it. Beware that some big-brand honeys have been found to be contaminated or even contain high fructose corn syrup. Liquid honey is easiest to use in herbal honey infusions, while thicker honey can be more manageable for first aid and wound care.

Oils. You can use olive oil for most purposes, though in some instances you'll want a lighter oil, such as grapeseed or almond, or a thicker oil such as shea butter or cocoa butter. You can even use animal-derived oils, such as lard, tallow, or lanolin.

Beeswax. Salves require wax to thicken them. You can buy beeswax in rounds or chunks and cut it down for each use. You can also buy beeswax pellets, which can be easier to work with.

Witch hazel extract. Look for a witch hazel extract made without alcohol, as this is most versatile—especially for first aid or wound care.

Rose water. Traditionally used for skin care, though also as a food ingredient. Rose water from the "ethnic foods" section of the grocery store is just as good as the higher-priced stuff in the health and beauty aisle.

Sea salt and Epsom salts. For baths and soaks as well as nasal sprays and gargles, a bit of salt improves the medicine.

Gelatin capsules. The "00" size is most frequently used when working with herbal powders to make homemade herb capsules.

Safety Precautions and Best Practices

Making and working with herbal remedies is very safe. Still, it's important to keep a few common-sense guidelines in mind to ensure you get the most out of your ingredients and your time.

Safety Tips

Label everything. If you don't know what you're taking, you can't be sure it's safe. Include details about all the ingredients in the remedy, as well as the date it was made.

Start small. Begin with small test batches and small doses when working with a new remedy. You can always scale up or take more later, but if an herb or preparation doesn't agree with you, it's best to discover that with a small amount.

Be cautious with pharmaceuticals. Herbs and pharmaceutical drugs (including both prescription and over-the-counter medications) can interact in many ways. Sometimes this is beneficial —positive herb-drug interactions may allow someone to reduce the dose of a drug or minimize its side effects—but it is a complicated subject and should be handled very carefully.

We identify the major interactions to watch for in the notes that accompany each remedy, but it's always best to consult with a practicing herbalist familiar with this topic, or your health care provider, especially if multiple drugs are taken simultaneously.

Best Practices

Use your senses. *Look* at the herbs you're working with, and your finished product. Check for mold in your jar of infused oil, check for bits of packaging material in your shipment of dried herbs. *Smell and taste* your herbs and remedies to get a sense of their potency, and dose accordingly.

Make only what you need. If you get great results from a particular remedy and you want to have it on hand every day, great—go for it. But no one needs a gallon of nasal spray solution, and it'll go bad before you even get around to using it. Make only those remedies you need, and only as much as you need.

Begin with what's abundant. In this book, we focus on herbs that are highly prevalent in the wild or grown commercially on a large scale. As you branch out into working with other plants, keep your focus on those that are local to you, and neither at risk nor endangered. Don't be tricked into thinking a rare, exotic herb will be the only one to solve your problem—it's vanishingly rare for that to be true.

Get the herb to the tissue. Herbs need to be in contact with the affected tissue to help it. We can't always just drink some herbal tea and get good results. Choose a delivery method that helps your herbs get where they need to act.

A few examples: If you're working with a respiratory problem, go with a steam; if you've got something on the skin, apply a soak or poultice; if it's trouble in the lower intestine, swallow some powder so it's intact when it gets down there.

Infusions

If you think of making tea, you probably picture an infusion. It's the simplest, most fundamental way to work with herbs, and is our preferred method in most circumstances. Infusions can be prepared in a variety of ways, but these are the most common:

Hot infusion. Like using a tea bag, a short, hot infusion means pouring boiling water on your herbs, letting them steep for a few minutes, and drinking as soon as tolerably cool. This method is best for herbs with aromatic or volatile constituents, which will evaporate if left to infuse too long.

Cold infusion. This method is used for demulcent, or mucilaginous, herbs, such as marshmallow—those that increase the water's viscosity as they infuse, rendering it first "velvety," then slimy. This only happens in cold water; hot water doesn't release the constituents responsible for this effect.

Long infusion. When trying to extract mineral content from nutritive herbs such as nettle, a long infusion is required. When done in a tightly sealed jar, this method also allows us to combine the quick-release aromatic constituents of one herb with the slow-release mucilage from another, as the initially hot water cools over time.

Administration and Dosage Guidelines

Infusions are generally drunk as they are. They may also serve as an ingredient in another remedy (bath, soak, compress, syrup, lotion, etc.). Each infused herb or formula has its own dosage ranges, but, for most in this book, it is normal to drink a quart of infusion daily, sometimes more.

Shelf Life and Storage Guidelines

Dry herbs blended for an infusion can keep for years if they're stored in airtight containers. Once water is added, infusions are generally only good for 1 or 2 days; if kept refrigerated, this could extend to 3 days. Trust your tongue: If the tea tastes "skunky" or otherwise off, best to make a new batch.

Necessary Tools, Equipment, or Ingredients

- Herbs
- Water
- Teacup, teapot, mason jar, French press, or other container
- Mesh strainer

Preparing Remedies: Step-by-Step Instructions

1. Unless otherwise specified, use 2 to 3 tablespoons of herbs per quart of water. (If making only a single cup of tea, use 1 to 3 teaspoons of herbs.)

2. Combine the herbs with the water and let steep:

   Hot infusion. Pour boiling water over the herbs, cover, and steep for 20 minutes or until cool enough to drink.

   Cold infusion. Pour cold or room-temperature water over the herbs and steep for 4 to 8 hours.

   Long infusion. Pour boiling water over the herbs, cover tightly, and steep for 4 to 8 hours or overnight.

3. Once the herbs have steeped, you may strain the liquid and compost the *marc* (leftover herb material).

Pros

Easy to make. Hot water, herbs, and a container are all you need.

Versatile. Infusions can be employed in a variety of ways, depending on need.

Potent. Each infusion method extracts a broad spectrum of constituents from the herbs, giving a good reflection of their full potential.

Hydrating. Drinking enough water is important for good health; infusions count as water intake.

Cons

Taken in quantity. When you drink an infusion, you need at least a teacup or two for beneficial effects. Not all herbs taste good, and some can be unpleasant to drink in that quantity.

Short shelf life. Once made, consume infusions promptly.

Additional Considerations

A press pot is a handy way to make infusions—you can steep them inside for a long time while still keeping them hot. For long infusions, you can also use a drip coffee maker: Put the herbs into the carafe (not the filter basket), turn it on, and let the water drip down onto them. They'll stay warm on the hot plate, shortening the amount of time you need to infuse them. (If it was ever used for coffee, though, this'll make your tea taste like it.)

Decoctions

Another method of making tea, decoctions are necessary when working with roots, barks, seeds, and other hard or woody plant parts. These require more time exposed to high heat to release their benefits into the water.

Administration and Dosage Guidelines

Like infusions, decoctions are generally drunk as they are. They may also serve as an ingredient in another remedy (bath, soak, compress, syrup, lotion, etc.). Each decoction has its own dosage range depending on the herbs used, but, for most in this book, it is normal to drink two cups to a quart of decoction daily.

Shelf Life and Storage Guidelines

Dry herbs blended for a decoction formula can keep for years if they're stored in airtight containers. Once water is added, decoctions are generally only good for 1 or 2 days at room temperature; if kept refrigerated, this could extend to 3 days.

Necessary Tools, Equipment, or Ingredients

- Herbs
- Water
- Quart- to gallon-size pot
- Mesh strainer

Preparing Remedies: Step-by-Step Instructions

1. Unless otherwise specified, use 2 to 4 tablespoons of herbs per quart of water.

2. Put the herbs and water in a lidded pot on the stove, cover, and bring to a boil.

3. Once boiling, reduce the heat and simmer for 20 minutes to 1 hour, stirring occasionally.

4. Strain the liquid for consumption and compost the marc.

5. Or, you may also choose to ladle out a teacupful at a time, leaving the water and marc in the pot until you strain off the last cup.

Pros

Easy to make. A stove, herbs, water, and a good pot are all you need.

Versatile. Decoctions can be employed in a variety of ways, depending on need.

Potent. Decoctions can be quite potent, as the simmering process extracts a majority of the herbs' available constituents.

Hydrating. Decoctions count as water intake.

Cons

Take time to make. Decoctions require a bit of time to prepare, so they're not great for resolving something quickly, like a bee sting or an asthma attack.

Taken in quantity. When you drink a decoction, you need at least a teacup or two for beneficial effects. Not all herbs taste good, and some can be unpleasant to drink in that quantity.

Short shelf life. Once made, consume decoctions promptly.

Additional Considerations

Generally, each herb is either infused or decocted, depending on what kind of plant part it is:

* Leaves, flowers, and stems are usually **infused**.
* Roots, seeds, and barks are usually **decocted**.

If you want to include both types of herb material in one drink, first decoct your hard herb parts. Then strain that liquid while still hot, and add your lighter plant bits to it for infusion. Strain one more time and it's ready to drink.

Sometimes decoctions are made in an open pot, allowing evaporation to reduce the volume of water. This concentrates the decoction's strength. For example, Elderberry Syrup—the herbs are first decocted, the liquid is reduced to half, and then it is mixed with honey.

Steams

Herbal steams are excellent for addressing issues in the lungs and sinuses, the face, and eyes. The evaporating steam carries light chemicals from the herbs, including some with antimicrobial, anti-inflammatory, relaxant, and immune-stimulating effects. These get into direct contact with the respiratory tract and skin, exerting their effects strongly.

Administration and Dosage Guidelines

Administer a steam whenever you want to stimulate the surface or respiratory tissues with moist heat.

For acute illness, it's best to steam at least twice a day. For ongoing skin or respiratory support, once a day is sufficient.

Shelf Life and Storage Guidelines

Steams are made on an as-needed basis; they are not stored.

Necessary Tools, Equipment, or Ingredients

* Herbs
* Water
* Gallon-size or larger pot
* Towel or blanket

Preparing Remedies: Step-by-Step Instructions

1. On the stove, boil ½ to 1 gallon of water in a covered pot.

2. Once at a full boil, remove from the heat and place the pot on a heat-proof surface.

3. Make a tent by draping a blanket or towel over your head.

4. Remove the lid from the pot and add ¼ to ½ cup of your herb mixture to the water.

5. Position your face over the steam and remain there for 5 to 20 minutes, catching the steam with your tent.

6. For respiratory issues, inhale the steam as deeply as you can so the medicated steam gets deep into your lungs.

7. Keep a handkerchief nearby—the steam will clear your sinuses and make your nose run.

Pros

Delivers the medicine where it's needed. Particularly for antimicrobial effects, steam is the most direct method for getting the herbs in contact with the respiratory tract tissues.

Stimulating but soothing. The warmth and moisture of steams help activate immune function in the mucous membranes and at the same time relieve irritation and calm a cough or ease difficult breathing.

Cons

Takes time. Between preparation and execution, it can take at least 30 minutes to conduct a good, effective steam.

Not portable. Steams require some space and a stove to make effectively, so they're mostly done at home.

Additional Considerations

After steaming, you can use the leftover liquid—it's essentially a hot infusion. Drink it, soak your feet in it, soak a cloth and make a compress, or employ it in some other way so nothing is wasted. If nothing else, let it cool and feed it to your garden or houseplants— plants like tea, too.

You can also make a good steam using essential oils. Simply boil water and set up your steaming station as directed, but instead of adding dry herbs, tap in 10 to 30 drops of essential oil. (Do not drink the leftover liquid when done steaming; just pour it down a drain.)

Baths and Soaks

Bathing or soaking part of the body in an herbal tea is a great way to get the herbs in contact with the affected part. These are good for infected skin or wounds, burns, rashes, and all manner of topical troubles.

Administration and Dosage Guidelines

You might make a whole-body bath with herbs, or you may just soak a particular part (as with a footbath or sitz bath). Keeping the water as hot as tolerable is best, as this facilitates absorption of the herbal medicines. For most issues, it's effective to soak for 15 to 20 minutes, 1 to 3 times per day.

Shelf Life and Storage Guidelines

Baths and soaks are prepared on an as-needed basis; they are not stored.

Necessary Tools, Equipment, or Ingredients

- Herbs
- Water
- Salt (optional)
- Vinegar (optional)
- Bathtub, dish basin, or other soaking vessel

Preparing Remedies: Step-by-Step Instructions

1. Prepare the water extraction (infusion or decoction) of the herbs.

2. Pour the extraction into a dish basin or similar container. For a whole-body bath, fill the bathtub with hot water, and pour in the herbal tea (at least one full quart).

3. If using vinegar, salt, or additional water, add it now. Stir to incorporate and dissolve. Test the heat with your hand, and submerge the affected body part.

4. Soak for a minimum of 15 to 20 minutes.

Pros

Delivers the medicine where it's needed. Baths and soaks are great for skin conditions and wounds. They work quickly for topical issues where internal use would be very slow or ineffective.

Cons

Not everything fits. Some body parts don't fit well into a soaking vessel, or are hard to soak separately (shoulders, for example). Use a compress in those cases.

Takes time. Between preparation and execution, it can take at least 30 minutes to conduct an effective soak.

Not portable. Baths require space and privacy, so they're usually done at home.

Additional Considerations

If your town or city chlorinates its tap water, it is best to use a chlorine filter on the water you bathe or soak in. Inexpensive filters can be found online; we prefer ones that use vitamin C cartridges or tablets, as this takes care of chloramines as well.

Warm, moistened skin is more absorptive; after a good soak, follow up with salve or other topical applications. They'll work even better than usual.

Poultices and Compresses

A poultice is a mass of warm, wet plant matter applied directly to the skin or a wound. A compress is simply a tea-soaked cloth or bandage applied similarly. Used for similar functions as a bath or soak, these can be applied to a specific area more easily and precisely.

Administration and Dosage Guidelines

Once you have the poultice or compress in place, keep it there for 5 to 20 minutes. Repeat 1 to 3 times per day.

Shelf Life and Storage Guidelines

Poultices and compresses are prepared on an as-needed basis; they are not stored.

Necessary Tools, Equipment, or Ingredients

* Herbs
* Water
* Washcloth, rag, bandana, etc.
* Cheesecloth

Preparing Remedies: Step-by-Step Instructions

Start by gently cleaning the affected area.

1. **For a poultice:**

   a. Place 4 to 6 tablespoons of the herb mixture in a heat-proof dish.

   b. Pour boiling water over the herbs, just enough to fully saturate them—not enough so they're swimming. Let the herbs soak for about 5 minutes.

   c. Scoop the herbs out of the dish onto a piece of cheesecloth or a bandage and give it a squeeze (like you would a teabag when you take it out of the water).

   d. Apply the mass of herbs, warm and wet, to the affected area. (You may prefer to wrap the herbs in a layer or two of cheesecloth to keep them contained.)

   e. Cover with a cloth and keep in place for 5 to 20 minutes, then gently dry.

2. **For a compress:**

   a. Prepare the water extraction (infusion or decoction) of the herbs you'll be working with, and strain.

   b. Soak a cloth in the hot tea, holding it by a dry spot and allowing the cloth to cool in the air until hot but comfortable to the touch.

   c. Lay the wet cloth over the affected area. Cover with a dry cloth.

   d. Get comfortable and let it soak in for 10 to 20 minutes.

3. Clean the area again, and bandage or cover if appropriate.

Pros

Delivers the medicine where it's needed. Poultices and compresses can be used to deliver herbal medicines to areas that are hard to soak. They work quickly for topical issues where internal use would be very slow or ineffective.

Soothing and stimulating. These preparations stimulate local circulation in the skin and underlying tissues, which helps speed healing. At the same time, they relax tension that prevents healthy, fluid movement.

Cons

Messy. It's easy to get herbs or tea all over yourself and your furniture when applying a poultice or compress. Lots of towels and secure wrapping help.

Takes time. Between preparation and execution, it can take at least 30 minutes to prepare and administer a poultice or compress.

Not portable. Poultices and compresses are usually only done at home.

Additional Considerations

Don't use the same compress cloth twice in one sitting—use a new cloth for each dip into the tea. (This is most critical when dealing with infected wounds, but make a habit of it in all situations.)

You may want to prepare a hot water bottle when setting up your poultice or compress, to lay on top and keep the application warm longer.

Be sure to clean the affected area both before and after using your compress and especially when using a poultice. Don't leave any little bits of herbal material on the irritated skin or in the wound.

Tinctures

Tinctures are among the most important methods of herbal medicine making you can learn, because of their potency, versatility, portability, and long shelf life. Fortunately, making a good tincture isn't much harder than making a nice cup of tea.

Administration and Dosage Guidelines

Tincture doses are measured by the dropperful, with the assumption that you're working from a dose bottle that is 1 to 4 fluid ounces in size and has a dropper top. Squeezing the dropper and allowing it to fill as much as possible makes 1 "dropperful," even though the entire glass dropper won't be filled to the top. Measured strictly, this will be about 1 milliliter of liquid per dropperful.

Most tinctures are taken in doses of 1 to 4 droppersful, 3 to 5 times per day.

If you don't have any dropper tops on hand, use a teaspoon. One teaspoon is equivalent to about 5 milliliters, so if the remedy calls for a dose of 2 to 4 droppersful, you can use ½ to 1 teaspoon and it'll be close enough.

Shelf Life and Storage Guidelines

Tinctures should be stored in colored glass bottles, or kept in a dark place, to prevent degradation from light exposure. For long-term storage, use a bottle with a flat cap rather than a dropper top—the rubber in the dropper will degrade over time if exposed to alcohol fumes.

If stored properly, tinctures will retain full potency for 5 to 10 years, or even longer.

Necessary Tools, Equipment, or Ingredients

- Herbs; if using fresh, let wilt for a half day or so spread out on brown paper bags or a clean tabletop (some water content will evaporate). Then chop or run through a blender before you put in the jar and add the alcohol.
- 80 or 100 proof (40 to 50 percent alcohol content) alcohol (vodka, brandy, or other)
- Mason jars, various sizes, for maceration
- Dose and storage bottles
- Strainers
- Funnels
- Labels

Preparing Remedies: Step-by-Step Instructions

1. Fill a mason jar half to three-fourths full with the herb you want to tincture. If using roots, which tend to swell in liquid, stay on the half-full side; if using leaves or flowers, fill to the three-fourths mark.

2. Fill the jar to the top with alcohol. Close securely and label the jar, including the date you started ("Chamomile tincture in vodka, 50 percent alcohol, 1/3/2018").

3. Macerate (allow the herbs to infuse in the alcohol) for 4 weeks. Shake the bottle every day or so to encourage maximum

constituent release. Otherwise, keep in a cool, dark place.

4. Strain, re-bottle in colored glass, and add the finish date to the label.

Pros

Small amounts are effective. For herbs with unappealing flavors, you can get an effective dose without having to drink a pot of tea.

Versatile. Tinctures can be taken as they are, blended into formulas, or mixed with other ingredients, as in elixirs and liniments.

Portable. Tincture dose bottles can be carried easily in a bag or stashed in a drawer at work, and are ready to take as soon as you need them.

Long shelf life. Tinctures can last decades if properly stored.

Cons

Contain alcohol. Tinctures cannot be used by those who cannot consume alcohol (e.g., due to liver problems, being a recovering alcoholic, religious reasons, etc.).

Preparation time. Tinctures made by maceration take at least 2 weeks, usually 1 month, to be ready. You'll have to plan ahead.

Additional Considerations

There is some variation in tincture-making processes, and more precise methods use weights and measures to arrive at a standardized ratio of plant matter to menstruum (the solvent), often seen on a tincture bottle as a ratio, such as 1:5, indicating that each 5 milliliters of tincture carries the equivalent of 1 gram of herb material. The simple maceration method described here will suffice in most situations.

You can use any alcohol you like for tincturing. A student of ours made an excellent catnip tincture in tequila, and we tincture herbs intended for the urinary system in gin because it already contains juniper, which is a urinary antiseptic herb.

Some plants require more alcohol, some more water. The vast majority of plants are fine to tincture in vodka or brandy (40 to 50 percent alcohol). When extracting resins, consider using grain alcohol (95 percent). When extracting mucilages, use water with just enough alcohol to prevent molding (20 percent of the total). For shelf-stable preservation, 20 percent alcohol is the minimum.

You can tincture herbal powders; they just require a lot more shaking to extract well and are a bit more difficult to strain at the end.

Practically speaking, you'll make larger amounts (pints to quarts) of individual plant tinctures, then blend them together in small amounts (2 to 8 fluid ounces) of formulas. As time goes on, you may find a lot of help from a particular formula and want to have more on hand, but wait until you've worked through your first few ounces (to make sure you like it or know better how much you need) before you do that.

It's also okay to tincture more than one plant together right from the start, rather than tincturing them all individually and then blending the tinctures.

Herb-Infused Vinegars

Vinegar is a useful menstruum (solvent) for herbal extracts. Its acidity helps draw out certain constituents called alkaloids, which are often some of the most potent chemicals in an herb. It also helps dissolve plant cell walls and release mineral content. Apple cider vinegar is standard in these preparations.

Administration and Dosage Guidelines

Herbal vinegars may be useful as remedies in their own right, such as Fire Cider, or they may be combined with honey to make an oxymel (see <u>here</u>).

    Herb-infused vinegars are frequently taken in doses of ½ to 1 fluid ounce at a time.

Shelf Life and Storage Guidelines

Like tinctures, store herbal vinegars in dark, light-blocking glass bottles in a cool, dry place. Vinegars will last at least 6 months (and up to several years).

Necessary Tools, Equipment, or Ingredients

- Herbs; if using fresh, let wilt for a half day or so spread out on brown paper bags or a clean tabletop (some water content will evaporate). Then chop or run through a blender before you put in the jar and add the vinegar.
- Apple cider vinegar
- Mason jars, various sizes, for maceration
- Dose and storage bottles
- Strainers
- Funnels
- Labels

Preparing Remedies: Step-by-Step Instructions

1. Fill a mason jar half to three-fourths full with the herb you want to extract. If using roots, which tend to swell in liquid, stay on the half-full side; if using leaves or flowers, fill to the three-fourths mark.

2. Fill the jar to the top with apple cider vinegar.

3. If using a mason jar with a metal lid, insert a piece of wax paper under the jar lid before screwing down the ring. The vinegar fumes will degrade the coating on the underside of the jar lids. If you like, use plastic lids instead to avoid this issue.

4. Close securely and label the jar, including the date you started ("Nettle-infused vinegar, 1/3/2018").

5. Macerate (allow the herbs to infuse in the vinegar) for 4 weeks. Shake the bottle every day or so to encourage maximum constituent release. Otherwise, keep in a cool, dark place.

6. Strain, re-bottle in colored glass, and add the finish date to the label.

Pros

Vinegar's innate benefits. Taken internally, vinegar stimulates digestion and can help with blood sugar control. Topically, it has antimicrobial, antifungal, and anti-inflammatory effects. Adding herbs enhances these further.

No alcohol. Vinegar extracts can be given in place of tinctures for those who can't consume alcohol, though they're not quite as strong.

Cons

The acidity. For some people who have heartburn or ulcers, vinegar's acidity can be too irritating to tissues already tender and inflamed.

Preparation time. Infused vinegars take at least 2 to 4 weeks to prepare.

Additional Considerations

Always use a high-quality, preferably raw, apple cider vinegar—not distilled white vinegar. Raw apple cider vinegar has probiotic content that can be helpful in some circumstances, like when making a digestive formula as a vinegar extract.

Herb-Infused Honeys

Herbal honeys are profoundly medicinal—and they taste great. When herbs are infused into honey, the honey absorbs all the water-soluble components of the herb and all the volatiles (essential oils), as well. This yields an excellent extraction of the herb's complex chemistry and preserves it very well.

Administration and Dosage Guidelines

For internal use, herb-infused honeys can be taken as they are. More often, though, they're used as ingredients in composite remedies, such as elixirs, oxymels, or syrups. Herbal honeys are also applied topically for skin blemishes, wounds, burns, etc.

If taken straight up, teaspoon and tablespoon doses of herb-infused honey will deliver an effective dose of herbal constituents.

Shelf Life and Storage Guidelines

Finished herbal honeys should be stored in sealed glass jars, away from light and heat. They will retain their potency for many years.

Necessary Tools, Equipment, or Ingredients

* Fresh herbs
* Honey
* Wide-mouth jars
* Wire mesh strainer
* Labels

Preparing Remedies: Step-by-Step Instructions

1. Coarsely chop your fresh herbs and allow them to wilt for a few hours before infusing.

2. Put your herbs into a wide-mouth jar and fill half to three-fourths full.

3. If the honey you're working with is a liquid consistency, simply pour it into the jar up to the shoulder. If it's solid or semi-solid, gently warm it to get it runny—set the honey jar in a pot of hot (not boiling) water for 10 to 30 minutes. The honey will soften and become easier to pour.

4. Using a chopstick or spoon, stir and work the herbs around in the honey.

5. Close securely and label the jar with the date and the herbs used.

6. Place in a warm area (like on top of the refrigerator) and leave to macerate for 4 weeks.

7. Gently warm the closed jar in a pot of hot water until the honey has a liquid consistency, then strain into a new jar. Press the marc against the strainer to express as much honey as you can.

8. Label the finished jar of infused honey and store in a cool, dark place.

Pros

Honey's innate benefits. Even before infusing with herbs, honey is an excellent wound healer and antimicrobial agent with a long history of use.

Long shelf life. Honey is an incredible preservative. You can expect your infused honey to last for years and retain its effects.

Delicious. Getting someone to take a honey medicine never seems to require much bargaining, even with kids and those who have picky palates.

Cons

Sweet means sugar. Herbal honeys taken alone are not ideal for those with insulin resistance, diabetes, or other blood sugar regulation problems. (When mixed into an oxymel or elixir, though, this concern is minimal.)

Potential fermentation. Because we're infusing fresh herbs into honey, there's the possibility that the water content of the herbs will thin out the honey, making it sufficiently liquid to allow it to ferment spontaneously.

Preparation time. Infused honeys take 1 month or more to prepare.

Additional Considerations

Choose local honey whenever possible. Aside from supporting local beekeepers (and local bees), honey made in your area will help you acclimate to pollen and reduce seasonal allergies.

Raw, unfiltered, unpasteurized honey has the most medicinal efficacy, but don't worry too much if you can't find this in your area. Most studies on honey as a wound dressing have been done with processed and irradiated honey, and it's still very effective.

Do be aware that some "honeys" sold in stores have been found to contain high fructose corn syrup or other adulterants. Make sure your honey is actually honey!

Syrups

Syrups are often made using sugar, but we vastly prefer to work with honey because of its innate benefits (see here). While the finished product is not shelf stable, it keeps well refrigerated.

Administration and Dosage Guidelines

Syrups are taken by the teaspoon or tablespoon, straight up, or stirred into tea.

Shelf Life and Storage Guidelines

Kept refrigerated, a honey-based syrup will last for several months. Light-blocking storage bottles are best, but as the syrup will be in the dark refrigerator most of the time, they're not as critical as they are for tinctures.

Necessary Tools, Equipment, or Ingredients

- Herbs
- Water
- Pot, for decoction
- Wire mesh strainers
- Honey, plain or herb infused
- Funnels
- Storage bottles
- Labels

Preparing Remedies: Step-by-Step Instructions

1. Prepare a tea with your herbs and water—either an extra-strong infusion (use twice as much herb as usual) or a concentrated decoction. If making a decoction, allow the water to evaporate as it simmers, reducing the original volume of water to half or one-fourth the original amount.

2. Strain and combine the concentrated decoction with an equal amount of honey, warming gently as you stir to mix thoroughly.

3. Bottle, label, and refrigerate.

Pros

Delicious. Syrups are appealing to almost everyone because of their sweetness.

Multiple extractions. If you use an herb-infused honey, your syrup contains both honey and water extracts of herbs, maximizing the extraction of a broad array of plant chemicals.

Cons

Needs refrigeration. This makes the syrups less portable.

Potential for mold. Always examine your syrup when you open the jar to take a dose. If there's any sign of mold growth on the surface, discard it and make a new batch.

Additional Considerations

Some recipes for herbal syrups call for sugar, as this creates a shelf-stable product. Instead of adding honey, you would add twice as much sugar as you have tea—so, for 4 cups of tea add 8 cups of sugar. That's a lot of sugar—the major reason we don't prefer this method.

You can make a honey syrup shelf stable by adding an equal amount of tincture to your syrup once it's made. So, for 2 cups of finished syrup, add 2 cups of tincture. This could be the same herb(s) used in your syrup—again increasing the range of constituents extracted—or complementary plants, creating a synergistic formula.

Oxymels and Elixirs

An oxymel is a blend of vinegar and honey. The vinegar releases minerals from the herbs, whereas alcohol really doesn't, and offers a substitute for those who avoid or don't want to use alcohol. "Plain" oxymel is an ancient remedy that lends particular support to the digestive and respiratory systems.

An elixir, broadly speaking, is a tincture combined with any sweetener. Honey is our preferred sweetener, though occasionally we use maple syrup or molasses, or even just tincture our herbs in a sweet liqueur (like rose petals steeped in St. Germain elderflower liqueur).

Administration and Dosage Guidelines

Elixirs and oxymels are generally taken by the dropperful, like tinctures, though they can also be taken in teaspoon or even tablespoon doses, as they are somewhat less potent than straight tinctures.

Shelf Life and Storage Guidelines

Oxymels and elixirs should be stored just like tinctures, in amber or blue glass bottles kept in a cool, dry place. Use flat caps on storage bottles and dropper tops on dose bottles. They'll keep for 6 to 12 months.

Necessary Tools, Equipment, or Ingredients

- Alcohol or vinegar
- Honey
- Mason jars, various sizes, for maceration
- Dose and storage bottles
- Wire mesh strainers
- Funnels
- Labels

Preparing Remedies: Step-by-Step Instructions

1. You can blend tinctures or vinegars you've already made with honey (either plain or herb infused) to create your oxymel or elixir, or you can macerate your herbs in the honey and alcohol, or honey and vinegar, at the same time.

2. If you're macerating the herbs in honey and alcohol or vinegar at the same time, proceed as if making a tincture (see here) or herb-infused vinegar (see here), but fill the jar only halfway with one of those liquids. Then add honey to fill the rest of the way.

3. Cover, label, and macerate for 4 weeks.

4. Strain, bottle, and label.

Pros

Effective in small doses. Oxymels and elixirs exert noticeable effects in dropperful and teaspoon amounts.

Portable. These are shelf stable and can be easily carried in a pocket or handbag.

Good tincture substitute. Oxymels are preferred for those who can't consume alcohol, can be nearly as potent as tinctures, and extract a broad range of constituents; they're better than infused vinegar alone.

Cons

Preparation time. If you're starting from scratch, it'll be 1 month or so before your oxymel or elixir is ready to use. (If you're blending premade tinctures, infused vinegars, and honeys, this isn't a problem.)

Additional Considerations

For elixirs: You might use equal parts honey and alcohol as described previously, or you might use as little as 1:3 (that is, the final mix will be one-fourth honey and three-fourths alcohol). You could include less honey, but below that ratio you'll start to lose the honey's medicinal contributions (separate from the herbs carried in it).

For oxymels: Equal parts honey and vinegar is standard, but a 1:5 ratio (1 part honey and 5 parts vinegar) will still get good effects.

Feel free to combine alcohol, vinegar, and honey all in one.

Herb-Infused Oils

Oils extract a very different set of chemical constituents from herbs than do water or alcohol. Infused oils *can* be consumed—think of a nice rosemary-infused olive oil with vinegar on a salad—though most often we work with them in topical preparations.

Administration and Dosage Guidelines

Infused oils may be employed directly as massage oil, conveying their effects into the skin and underlying tissues, or mixed with other ingredients to make a liniment (see here) or lotion (see here). If you melt wax into an oil and let it cool and harden, you've made a salve (see here).

For most purposes, apply the infused oil liberally to the affected area, 1 to 5 times per day. Massage it into the tissue as much as possible; don't just wipe it over the surface. Work it in for a few solid minutes to encourage absorption and get the best effects.

Shelf Life and Storage Guidelines

Herb-infused oils should be stored in dark, light-blocking bottles in a cool, dry place. They will retain their potency for about 1 year if stored well.

Necessary Tools, Equipment, or Ingredients

- Herbs, fresh or dried
- Oil: olive, coconut, grapeseed, almond, etc.
- Oven-safe dish
- Mason jars, various sizes, for maceration
- Wire mesh strainers
- Cheesecloth
- Funnels
- Storage bottles

Preparing Remedies: Step-by-Step Instructions

When working with **fresh herbs**, we use a heat method, which allows the water to evaporate and helps prevent mold:

1. Chop the herbs coarsely and place in an oven-safe dish. Pour in enough oil so the herbs are submerged.

2. Put the dish in the oven and turn it to its lowest setting—ideally, 180°F or lower. If your oven doesn't go that low, set up a double boiler on the stove, use a simmer burner or hot plate, or use the "warm" (not "low") setting on a slow cooker.

3. Leave the herbs and oil exposed to heat for 8 to 12 hours. This doesn't have to be consecutive—you can turn the oven on for a few hours, then turn it off, as long as the total heating time is completed within 3 days.

4. Strain the oil and wrap the marc in cheesecloth. Squeeze out the last drops of oil from the marc.

5. Bottle in light-blocking glass and label. Use within 1 year.

When working with **dried herbs**, you may use the same heat method, or this no-heat method:

1. Fill a mason jar half to three-fourths full with the herbs you want to infuse.

2. Pour in enough oil to fill the jar. Cover and label.

3. Allow to macerate for 4 weeks.

4. Strain and wrap the marc in cheesecloth. Squeeze to express the last drops of infused oil from the marc.

5. Bottle in light-blocking glass and label. Use within 1 year.

Pros

Great for topical needs. Herbal oils are soothing, restorative, and hydrating to the skin. They also help herbal constituents penetrate into the tissue to do their work.

Innate benefits of oils. Each oil has its own beneficial qualities. Coconut oil is antifungal, olive oil is extra moistening and highly anti-inflammatory. Remember that the menstruum matters at least as much as the herbs we put into it.

Cons

Potential for mold. Examine your oil at least once a day while infusing. If there's any sign of mold growth on the surface, you can usually skim this off with a spoon without losing the entire batch. If there's mold growth at the bottom of the jar, though, the batch is lost. This is primarily a problem when infusing oil with fresh herbs and is the reason we use the heat method.

Preparation time. A heat infusion can be ready in 1 or 2 days, but a cold infusion takes at least 2 weeks.

Messy. Oils tend to leak out of their bottles, no matter how securely they're closed. If you keep some infused oil in a first aid kit or travel bag, enclose it in a resealable plastic bag as well.

Additional Considerations

Olive oil is the standard for infusions today, but only because it's so widely available. In the past, animal oils such as lard, tallow, and lanolin were the go-tos for these preparations. They're extremely well absorbed by human skin, and are worth consideration. For some purposes, it's preferable to use a lighter oil, like grapeseed or almond; other times, you want a thicker oil like cocoa butter, shea butter, or castor oil. Try different oils to see which you prefer. Whichever you choose, make sure it's made by a cold-press process. Cold-pressed oils are better quality than solvent-extracted oils, which are more likely to be rancid, plus there is solvent left in the oil, and many times those solvents, like hexane, are toxic.

    Note: An herb-infused oil is *not the same thing* as an essential oil. Essential oils are created by a distillation process and are extremely concentrated and potent. Never apply them directly to the skin without diluting in a carrier oil first, and do not take internally.

Liniments

We define a liniment as a blend of herb-infused oil with tincture, intended for topical use only. Some liniments also include essential oils. This combination of alcohol and oil allows us to get a full constituent extraction from the herbs, and it has both quick-acting and slow-release qualities in one.

Administration and Dosage Guidelines

When applying a liniment, massage it in until your hands no longer feel oily. Work the liniment into the tissue; don't just lightly rub it onto the surface.

Liniments should be applied 3 to 5 times per day, or more as needed.

Shelf Life and Storage Guidelines

It's better to store liniments in bottles with flat caps rather than dropper tops, as the oil can degrade the rubber on exposure. Simply tip a little into your palm when you want to use it.

Liniments are shelf stable and will retain potency for at least 1 year.

Necessary Tools, Equipment, or Ingredients

- Tinctures
- Infused oils
- Essential oil (optional)
- Funnels
- Bottles and caps
- Labels

Preparing Remedies: Step-by-Step Instructions

1. In your storage bottle, combine the tincture and infused oil.

2. If using essential oils, add at a ratio of 10 to 30 drops of essential oil per ounce of liniment.

3. Cap the bottle and label it, including *Shake well before each use.*

Pros

Double action. The tincture is rapidly absorbed and begins to work quickly, while the oil is absorbed more slowly and releases its medicine over time.

Safe essential oil use. Essential oils disperse nicely in a liniment, making this a safe way to work with them for topical purposes.

Cons

Messy. While not quite as troublesome as simple infused oils, liniments have a tendency to leak from their bottles. If you travel with a liniment, enclose the bottle in a resealable plastic bag.

Additional Considerations

Some herbalists define a liniment as a tincture made in rubbing alcohol or another substance that cannot be consumed, intended for topical use only.

Salves

A salve is an herb-infused oil with beeswax melted into it. Once cooled, it assumes a consistency somewhere between petroleum jelly and hard lip balm, depending on the amount of wax added and the ambient temperature.

Administration and Dosage Guidelines

Apply a liberal amount of salve to the affected area at least twice a day. Salves are best applied when the skin is hydrated and the pores are open, like after a shower or a soak.

Shelf Life and Storage Guidelines

Salves can be stored in glass jars, metal tins, or nonreactive plastic containers. Choose wide-mouth vessels that are not too deep, so you can reach to the bottom easily.

Salves are very stable, but should be used within 1 year for best potency.

Necessary Tools, Equipment, or Ingredients

- Herb-infused oil
- Beeswax, chopped, grated, or pellets; 1 ounce of wax for every 6 to 8 fluid ounces of oil
- Essential oil (optional)
- Small pot
- Shot glass
- Storage vessels
- Labels

Preparing Remedies: Step-by-Step Instructions

1. In a small pot over low heat, warm the oil gently and slowly—do not boil.

2. Add the beeswax. For a softer salve, use less wax. This is helpful when it will be applied to sensitive skin, or if used in cold climates. For a harder salve, use more wax. This is better if the salve will be used in hot climates or as lip balm.

3. Stir continuously until the wax melts.

4. Spoon some wax into a shot glass and freeze for a few minutes; it will set to its finished hardness. Take it out and test it with your finger to see if it is the consistency you want.

5. Add more wax to the pot if you want to harden the salve; add more oil if you want to soften it.

6. Add the essential oil (if using):
   - If you're pouring the hot salve into a single storage vessel, add the essential oil after doing so, stir quickly, and close the vessel so the essential oil does not evaporate.
   - If you're pouring the hot salve into multiple small vessels, add the essential oil before pouring, stir quickly, pour, and close the vessels immediately.
7. Label your vessels.

Pros

Portable. Salve is a good way to take a messy oil infusion and make it much more manageable.

Cons

Not for use on wet or open wounds. Salves should not be used on a fresh burn, weeping rash, open lacerations, or puncture wounds. The oil and wax form a seal that prevents airflow and can allow bacteria to grow in the wound. In the case of a burn, that seal prevents heat from dispersing. Use poultices or compresses until the wound closes up and dries out, and for a burn, until the skin begins to itch.

Additional Considerations

Clean your pot and utensils with paper towels, newsprint, or a dishrag while the salve is still hot and liquid. If it sets, use very hot water to melt it and wash it away.

You can buy empty tubes and pour hot salve directly into them to make your own lip balm.

Lotions

Lotions are what you get when oil and water mix. The trick is finding a way to keep them in suspension. Most instructions for making lotions call for water and herb-infused oils, but this yields a very thin, runny lotion that is more likely to separate. We find that working with salve instead of oils makes a thicker lotion more likely to stay mixed.

If you prefer thick lotions, use salve. If you prefer thin lotions, use oil. If you prefer something in between, use half salve and half oil.

Administration and Dosage Guidelines

Lotions are used topically for dry conditions, such as eczema and dermatitis. You can use them any time as part of your daily skin care routine. Lotions are excellent for later-stage healing of burns.

Apply lotions frequently for best results—2 to 4 times daily, depending on the issue.

Shelf Life and Storage Guidelines

Lotions should be used within 1 to 3 months. If you live in a hot climate, keep them refrigerated.

Necessary Tools, Equipment, or Ingredients

- Rose water, nonalcoholic witch hazel extract, tea, or water
- Herbal salve or herb-infused oil
- Blender
- Storage container
- Labels

Preparing Remedies: Step-by-Step Instructions

1. Make sure all ingredients are at room temperature—if any are warmer or cooler than the others, they may not emulsify.

2. Measure equal amounts of salve and water (plain water, tea, rose water, a water-based witch hazel extract, etc.)—no more than 1 cup each. (Blenders can usually handle 1½ to 2 cups of lotion total.)

3. Put the water in the blender and blend for 1 to 2 minutes until frothy.

4. Use a fork to stir the salve to soften it. With the blender running, slowly add the salve, a forkful at a time. If using oil, slowly pour it into the blender. Continue to blend for a few minutes; it will form a suspension and your finished lotion.

5. Bottle the lotion, cap the bottle, and label it, including *Shake well before each use.* If your lotion separates, shaking temporarily re-emulsifies it.

Pros

Emollient. Soothing for dry skin conditions.

Can be applied to burns. Once the skin starts to itch, lotion can provide relief and can be made with herbs that speed new skin growth, such as calendula.

Homemade is better. You can add any scent you like, and you know there are no preservatives or chemicals.

Cons

Tricky to make. It may take a few tries to find the best ratio of water to salve or water to oil. If your lotion is too thick, next time add more water. If too thin, next time add more salve. It is okay to put a lotion back into the blender to add more water or salve/oil—experiment until you get it the way you like it. Keep good notes so you can reproduce it next time.

Short shelf life. Make lotion in small batches so you can use it all before it molds.

Additional Considerations

If you adjust the recipe to increase the yield, blend it in small batches so there is no more than 2 cups total in the blender at one time. Most blenders can't emulsify more than 1½ to 2 cups at a time.

Capsules

Teas, tinctures, vinegars, and all other "solvents" extract only some of the herbs' constituents, but in powder form, you get everything the herb has to offer. This makes powders a very effective form for taking herbs. You *can* simply stir powdered herbs into hot water, broth, or tea—it's not the most appealing prospect, though, especially if you don't like gritty textures. Most people prefer to encapsulate them instead.

The Capsule Machine is a handy, inexpensive, manual capsule-filling device that makes it *much* easier to make your own capsules. (Encapsulators can be purchased at herbal supply retailers; see Resources)

Administration and Dosage Guidelines

Capsules are pretty straightforward—just swallow them with lots of water or tea.

Doses vary depending on the herb involved, but are usually between 1 and 6 capsules taken 1 to 3 times daily.

Shelf Life and Storage Guidelines

Powdered herbs should be enclosed in airtight containers and kept away from heat and light.

Because powdering exposes so much more surface area, they don't stay potent as long as whole dried herbs do. Once ground, it's best to use the powdered herbs within 2 weeks, or 1 month at most. This isn't mitigated by encapsulating them—the clock still counts down. Order powders in small batches—or, even better, grind them fresh each time.

Necessary Tools, Equipment, or Ingredients

- Powdered herbs or dried herbs and herb grinder
- Capsules
- The Capsule Machine (optional, but extremely helpful)

Preparing Remedies: Step-by-Step Instructions

1. If starting with cut and sifted dried herbs, use an herb grinder to render the dried herbs into a powder.

2. Using The Capsule Machine (or lots of patience), fill the capsules with powder and close them up.

Pros

Full spectrum. With any powder-based preparation, you get all the water-, alcohol-, and fat-soluble constituents the herb has to offer.

Portable. Capsules are handy when traveling.

Deep delivery. Capsules dissolve as they move through the digestive system, releasing their herb material when they get to the stomach or small intestine. You can buy special *enteric-coated* capsules (which will not dissolve in the stomach) to reach even farther down, enabling you to target the large intestine.

Cons

Sometimes hard to swallow. The "00" size capsules are fairly large and can be difficult for some people to swallow. Smaller capsules can be used, but the amount of herb each delivers then also decreases.

Lots of capsules equals not much powder. It takes 3 to 4 capsules to equal 1 teaspoon of powdered herbs. For some herbs, you'll want to consume tablespoons of powder for strong effects; to get doses that high from capsules requires swallowing an unreasonable number.

Short shelf life. Whether homemade or store-bought, use capsules within 1 month. They are much less stable than other forms of herbal medicine.

Additional Considerations

Homemade capsules are simply powder in a shell. Commercial capsules could contain powder, but these days they're often made with a *dried liquid extract* instead. This means the herb was extracted in a liquid medium and dehydrated to produce a resinous concentrate. Commercial capsules can thus attain a much greater potency than homemade, so not as many are required to get a medicinal effect.

Honey Powder Pastes

Aside from capsules, there are other ways to take powdered herbs. A honey powder paste, or *electuary*, is a particularly nice way to take them, and it preserves the herb material very well, too.

Administration and Dosage Guidelines

You can stir the honey powder paste into tea or hot cereal, or just eat it off the spoon.

For medicinal effects, take 1 to 3 teaspoons 2 to 3 times per day.

Shelf Life and Storage Guidelines

You can store honey powder paste in a glass jar for a year or more. As with other herbal medicines, it is best to keep it away from heat and light.

Necessary Tools, Equipment, or Ingredients

* Powdered herbs (You can grind your own, but the texture will be grittier, so we recommend starting with store-bought powdered herbs.)

- Honey
- Small, wide-mouth jars
- Small pot
- Water
- Stove or hot plate
- Labels

Preparing Remedies: Step-by-Step Instructions

1. Use a ratio of 1 part powdered herbs to 5 parts honey (for example, 2½ tablespoons powdered herbs to ¾ cup honey.)

1. Measure the honey and place it in a jar. It's best to use a squat, wide-mouth jar, as this will also be the container for your finished honey powder paste.

2. Warm the honey gently by placing the jar in a small pot of hot (not boiling) water on the stove or on a hot plate. (Don't let water get into the jar; keep the water level in the pot 1 to 2 inches below the jar's mouth.)

3. As the honey warms, it will transition suddenly to a thin, watery consistency. When this happens, remove it from the heat and stir the powdered herbs into the honey. Stir very, very well, making sure to break up any clumps of powder. Continue stirring for a few more minutes after you think it's all stirred in, so it will not separate or clump up. The paste will thicken as it cools and even more over time.

4. Close the jar and label it.

Pros

Long shelf life. When suspended in honey, the herb material is protected from oxidation and breakdown. Even powdered herbs will maintain their potency for years when they're preserved in honey.

Full spectrum. With any powder-based preparation, you get all the water-, alcohol-, and fat-soluble constituents the herb has to offer.

Delicious. While some don't like the grittiness of honey paste, the sweetness is very popular.

Cons

Sweet means sugar. Herbal honey powder pastes are not ideal for those with insulin resistance, diabetes, or other blood sugar regulation problems.

Gritty. Especially if you grind your own herbs at home, your paste may have a gritty texture that some don't enjoy. Commercially made powders are much finer and more consistent in texture, and yield a smoother paste.

Additional Considerations

In the Ayurveda medical tradition of India, it's common to make a similar preparation using ghee (clarified butterfat). It's not as sweet, but it can be employed in the same way as a honey powder paste.

Nut Butter Morsels

These tasty treats are a great way to introduce herbs to those who are skeptical about less familiar methods such as tincture or who just don't like to drink tea.

Administration and Dosage Guidelines

Nut butter morsels can be made simply for pleasure or as an intentional way to increase your intake of phytonutrients (beneficial plant chemicals).

Eating 1 to 4 daily equals a medicinal dose of herbal material.

Shelf Life and Storage Guidelines

Once made, keep nut butter morsels refrigerated in an airtight container; consume within 1 week.

Necessary Tools, Equipment, or Ingredients

- Powdered herbs
- Powdered spices or cocoa powder, for flavoring and coating
- Nut butter of choice
- Honey (optional)
- Unsweetened dehydrated shredded coconut (optional)
- Mixing bowl and spoons
- Airtight container

Preparing Remedies: Step-by-Step Instructions

A standard batch of nut butter morsels will use:

1 cup powdered herbs

¾ cup nut butter

½ cup honey (if using; if not, increase the nut butter to 1 cup)

¼ cup powdered spices (cinnamon, ginger, cayenne), unsweetened shredded coconut, or cocoa powder

1. In a medium bowl, combine the powdered herbs, nut butter, and honey (if using). Mix to form a thick dough.

2. Roll the dough into 20 to 24 (1-inch) balls.

3. Place the spices, cocoa, or coconut in a shallow dish and roll the balls to coat.

4. Refrigerate the morsels in an airtight container.

Pros

A good snack. With a decent amount of protein and very few carbohydrates (especially if you reduce or eliminate the honey), these make a great treat.

Full spectrum. With any powder-based preparation, you get all the water-, alcohol-, and fat-soluble constituents the herb has to offer.

Cons

Nut allergies. Try sunflower seed butter or tahini instead.

Short shelf life. Keep refrigerated and consume within 1 week.

Additional Considerations

If your morsels seem to "melt" or ooze out all their oil while in the refrigerator, it simply means you needed a little more powder in the mix. Including honey reduces the likelihood for this to happen, helping everything stick together.

Additional Herbal Preparations

A number of other simple herbal preparations are included with the ailments they help address in part 3. There, you'll find recipes for herbal mouthwash, skin toner, broth, wound wash, and more.

Due to costs involved, time to prepare, or difficulty of execution, we don't cover some remedies you may learn about as you continue to study herbalism. Here are a few worth mentioning:

- **Percolation tinctures.** Based on the same principle as a drip coffee maker, a percolation involves powdering the herb, moistening it, packing it into a glass cone, and dripping alcohol through it. The alcohol absorbs the herbal constituents and drips out the bottom as a finished tincture. This is a very handy procedure, as it gives you a completed tincture in just days, rather than weeks.

- **Double extractions.** For medicinal mushrooms and certain herbs, it's important to combine both alcohol and water extractions from the same plant matter.
- **Fluidextracts.** A fluidextract (yes, that's all one word) is a special kind of concentrated tincture made in a multi-step process. These were popular among the Eclectics, nineteenth-century herbal physicians who had status equivalent to "regular" doctors in their day—"regular" meaning standardized in training and equivalent to our medical doctors today.
- **Teapills.** Mostly associated with traditional Chinese medicine, teapills are made by condensing a decoction into a very thick liquid, blending it with herbal powder, and rolling the mixture into small, hard balls. Sometimes referred to as "patent medicines," referring not to a legal patent but to the standardization of classic formulas.

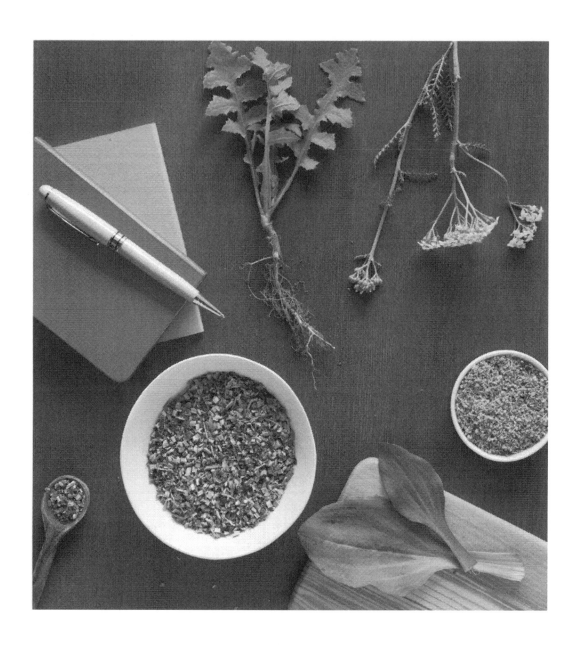

STEP FOUR
Work Safely with Herbal Medicine

Herbal medicine is very safe. It is rare for serious complications or negative effects to occur when working with herbal remedies. Even so, there's always potential for an herb to be incompatible with an individual person, for an allergic response to be triggered, or for the herb to be otherwise unhelpful. By following a few simple safety guidelines, we can avoid many of these issues, and the baseline safety of herbalism can be bolstered even further.

Dosages and Protocols

Herbs do not act the same way drugs do. This doesn't just mean herbs aren't as "strong" as drugs—they are not simply "weak drugs," as people often think. In contrast to the isolated chemical of a pharmaceutical, each herb is a complex of dozens or hundreds of different active constituents. These work synergistically, in the sense that various compounds work through independent mechanisms that all contribute to an observable effect.

There's also the importance of the body's response to the scent, flavor, and other sensory qualities of the herb or herbal remedy. When we smell an aromatic herb or taste a few drops of bitter tincture, there's a cascade of effects that moves through the entire body, one often far greater in magnitude than expected from the amount of chemicals that have been inhaled or ingested.

Because herbal medicines are so different in their mode of action from pharmaceutical medicines, their dosing amounts and protocols are quite different, too.

Dosage Recommendations

The most important thing to know about dosing herbal medicines is there is a great degree of individual variation. Each person's body will react slightly differently to each herb or remedy. View all dose recommendations in this book as a starting place only.

Each type of herbal preparation included in step 3 (starting here), and each remedy listed together with an ailment profile in part 3, includes baseline recommended doses. In our experience, people respond to anywhere from *one-fourth as much* to *four times as much* of these baseline doses.

Some things that might indicate you need a *higher* dose include:

* Cold or damp constitution (see here)
* Slow metabolism

- Larger body size
- Slow circulation
- Sluggish digestion
- Low sensitivity to pharmaceuticals

Some things that might indicate you need a *lower* dose include:
- Hot or dry constitution (see here)
- Fast metabolism
- Smaller body size
- Young or old age
- High sensitivity to pharmaceuticals
- Strong or multiple allergies or chemical sensitivities
- Impaired liver or kidney function

In the end, your direct experience with the herbs will be your best guide. Start on the low end of our recommended dosing ranges, and progress to higher doses if necessary.

Practical Protocols

Dose refers to the amount of an herb or remedy taken at one time. *Protocol* refers to the regimen or schedule according to which the doses are administered. When it comes to herbalism, they're equally important.

Very frequently, taking a single large dose of an herb is less effective than taking several smaller doses spread over the course of the day. In most cases, a single dose doesn't do it—herbs influence the body gently and work best when taken regularly over a period of time. Consistency and persistence win the day.

The herbs we cover in this book are almost all appropriate for long-term use: months, seasons, or years of consistent intake. (The exceptions are noted in the herb's profile and in any remedies which include it. *Ones to consider carefully are St. John's wort, uva-ursi, and wild lettuce.*)

"Long-term use" doesn't necessarily mean taking the same dose of the same herb every day for the rest of your life: We generally prefer to make a couple weeks' to a months' worth of a given formula, work with that until it's gone, and reassess. It may be appropriate to continue with the same herbs, or adjustments may be made to account for changes in your body that occur in the intervening time. An herb that played a major role when you first started working with it may shift to a support role later on, or vice versa. Sometimes it's appropriate to stop taking an herb for a period of time, to determine whether it's still necessary to keep your ailment at bay or if the need has passed. The point is to stay present, checking in regularly to ask, "Is this the right herb for me right now?"

We have very different constitutions—Ryn is 5'4" with a very fast metabolism and dry constitution; Katja is 5'11" with a slow metabolism and cold/damp constitution. It really shows in our herb dosing strategies. Although we both drink herbal tea all day long, when it comes to tinctures, Katja typically takes two to three times what Ryn does, or more. How can you decide? Feel it in your body! The herbs we include in this book are very safe to experiment with, so try several different doses and see what feels right for you.

For some purposes, particular timing strategies are required to produce the best effects. For instance, when giving herbs to support sleep, we often recommend "pulse dosing"—taking a small dose several times in the hour before bed, rather than taking a single large dose at bedtime. Another example is the use of bitters before meals as a digestive aid, which is most effective when taken 10 to 20 minutes before you eat. We've made notes about these kinds of details wherever relevant.

Aside from these ideas about timing and frequency, the idea of a health protocol also involves all interventions being undertaken to resolve an ailment or improve health. This could include rational changes to diet, sleep habits, movement patterns, and stress management strategies—the four pillars of good health. Remember, herbs work best when they're not working alone: Aligning your habits with your intentions for the herbal remedies will make for the most pervasive and lasting positive changes to health.

Tracking the Remedy's Effects

How can you know if an herb is working? And how can you tell what change made the difference?

The answer is simple and difficult at the same time, because it means developing an awareness of your body that doesn't necessarily come naturally. It's natural to notice when something is "wrong," but when everything is going well and you're feeling good, you're not always aware of it, or you may just think it's "normal." And when things do go wrong, you don't always have a clear understanding of why, because by the time you notice, the cause is already in the past. Developing this kind of awareness takes time— be patient!

One of the best tools we've found for keeping track of the effects of your work with herbs is journaling. Whether you use an app, a spreadsheet, or just a notebook and pen, it's handy to build a habit of noticing what's going on in your body and how you are responding to your environment.

We typically advise writing down everything that goes into your body: food, drink, supplements—anything you put in your mouth. This isn't about counting calories, so there's no need to *quantify* what goes in—just a simple list of ingredients is sufficient. Some other things that count as "input" are sleep, emotions, media, and personal and community events—anything you have to deal with emotionally, because those emotions often affect your physical health.

Then, keep track of everything that comes out, the "results," including things like a headache, constipation, or feeling run-down. Or maybe you felt energetic—anytime you notice any kind of result, make a note. You don't have to know why you feel that way, just make a note that you do.

Over time, you'll start to see patterns emerge. For example, one client who knew she had hypothyroidism started adding seaweed and nettles to her daily routine and started checking her temperature every morning when she woke up. Over the course of the next six to nine months, her baseline temperature increased by a whole degree, which showed she was experiencing a positive reaction in her thyroid health. Not all results take so long to see, but as you start to build new awareness about your states of health, you'll be more easily able to see your successes. Plus, over time, you'll build a very handy record: Let's imagine you have a certain time every year that is stressful at work. By keeping data, you will have a record of what worked best for you this year when that stressful time comes around again next year.

Sometimes, herbs don't have the effect you're looking for. That's okay! You should start to see enough results after a week to 10 days of consistent intake to know whether you're on the right track, even if everything isn't fully where you want it to be. If you're not getting the results you were hoping for, no problem: Try another tactic! Bodies are different, and what works best for one body isn't always what's best for another—that's why we list so many different herbs for each ailment. Be as detailed as possible as you think about your symptoms, because that will help you make more precise choices.

For example, we might both say we have "digestive upset"—but our bodies are very different. When Ryn has digestive upset, he's usually experiencing some nausea or heartburn-type feelings. When Katja has digestive upset, she's usually experiencing lower gut cramping and constipation. The same herb will not necessarily address both problems. This is a case where Ryn might reach for catnip, and Katja might reach for chamomile, because, even though we started with a problem that sounded the same, it turned out that the symptoms were actually different.

Helping the Herbs Go Down

It's true—some herbs are bitter. But many herbs are actually quite tasty, and making a delicious cup of tea is sometimes just as easy as pairing an herb you love, like ginger or peppermint, with a less-tasty herb you want to work with.

Other times, the bitter flavor is actually the point, such as when addressing many types of digestive issues. But just because it's bitter doesn't mean it can't be fun—blending bitters can create interesting new flavors. Mixing in herbs with strong flavors, such as fennel or angelica, can really spruce up an otherwise boring bitters blend, and when the flavor is interesting, we often discover the bitterness is not unpleasant!

We particularly love to blend herbs for stressful times, depression, or anxiety as elixirs—that extra bit of sweetness is a legitimate part of the medicine, especially when there are bitter emotions. Instead of thinking, "Oh, I should take that tincture . . . " an elixir is much more like a treat.

Herbs don't always have to be taken as a tea or tincture! Consider:

- Herbs in wine, chocolate, and cocktails
- Herbal honeys, elixirs, and oxymels
- Herbs in the bath and your skincare products
- Herbal sprays, incense, and "perfume" oils
- And, of course, herbs in your food!

Storing Herbal Medicines Well

Although you may have seen pictures of old homesteads with dried herbs hanging from the rafters, these days we have better storage methods to ensure your herbs stay fresh and last a long time.

Storage and Shelf Life Guide

The universal standard for storing basically any herbal product is mason jars. Whether dried herbs, tinctures, salves, elixirs—likely as not, herbalists put it in a mason jar. They come in all sizes; they're widely available, airtight, and inexpensive. The only thing they lack is color: dark-colored glass, such as amber or cobalt, prevents light from affecting the quality of the product you're storing. But those containers are more expensive, and, realistically, clear glass is fine as long as it's not in direct sunlight.

If stored in glass with a tight-fitting lid, you can expect dried herbs to last 1 to 5 years, and tinctures might last as long as 10 years. Oils and salves have a shorter shelf life, because oils go rancid eventually—they may only last 6 months to 1 year. Lotions have the shortest shelf life, because when you mix oil and water, you have a perfect medium for mold. Lotions may only last 1 to 3 months, but you can extend their life by refrigerating them.

The best way to detect if dried herbs or herbal products are still good is to use your senses: If it still smells strongly of the herb, if it still has bright vibrant color, if it still has potent flavor, it's still good.

TROUBLESHOOTING

I want to work with herbs, but I don't have much time.

Start with something very simple and build on it as you have time. There's no point in planning a complicated protocol you won't have time to implement. Just pick the thing that seems easiest and start there: Your success will build on itself!

A few simple tools can make the job faster and easier. A French press makes tea making and cleanup much quicker. Good-quality teabags are easy to take with you on the road. Tinctures can be stashed in your bag or in a pocket and don't require any preparation to use. Although it's great to have a nice, relaxing, slow cup of tea, what really matters is getting the herbs into you, whatever way is easiest.

I keep forgetting to bring my herbs to work with me.

Make sure you have a supply of the herbs you want to work with at home and at work, in a convenient form. That way, you don't have to remember to bring them with you every day. If you're planning to take a bitter tincture before meals, for example, keep a bottle of tincture at home and at work. To cover all your bases, have one in your bag or briefcase, too—then you know you're always prepared!

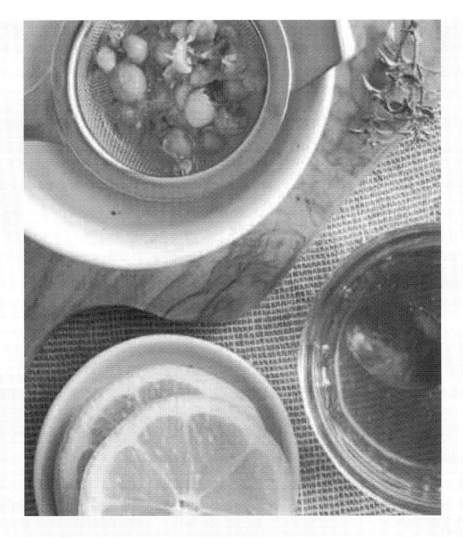

I don't like the flavor, so I just don't ever take it.

The best herb for you is the one you'll take—so, if you don't like the flavor of an herb you're working with, switch to something you *do* like. Even if it's not the perfect herb for the health changes you're trying to make, it *is* the perfect herb for helping you build new habits into your lifestyle. Once you develop the habit, you can switch up the herbs you're using—and you might be surprised to find your tastes have changed along the way. If all else fails, cover the flavor with something tastier, such as ginger or peppermint.

I tried, but it didn't work out. I don't think I can do this.

Learning new ways to keep your body strong and healthy can be challenging, but you don't have to get it right on the first try. Take it step by step; if one thing doesn't work, try something else. Start with the most enjoyable thing and work slowly. There's no one right way, so just incorporate what works best for you.

I'm nervous about taking herbs because I also take prescription medicines.

You don't have to take herbs internally to experience their benefits—consider putting herbs in your bath, in a foot soak, in a lotion, or other topical application. For example, if you have a headache but don't want to take herbs internally, you can put warm chamomile tea on a clean washcloth and lay it on your forehead while you rest for 10 to 15 minutes. This way, there is no concern about drug interactions, and you can still enjoy practicing herbalism. That being said, if you feel anxious about taking herbs, talk to your primary care provider or physician just to be safe.

I'm not sure where to get safe, good-quality herbs.

Check the Resources section for a list of our favorite herb suppliers. The suppliers listed all test their soil and/or their herbs to make sure there are no contaminants, grow their plants organically or ethically wild harvest them, and are mindful of their impact on the earth.

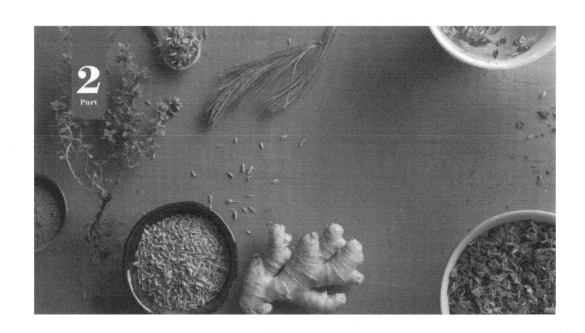

2
Part

Herb Profiles

In the following pages, you'll meet 35 herbs we think are most important for beginners. Many are probably growing in your neighborhood—we've chosen plants common in most areas of the United States. All these herbs are easy to find in commerce, whether online or at a local herb shop. They have low potential for allergic reactions or negative interactions with pharmaceuticals (and we've noted wherever either is a concern), so they're all quite safe to experiment with. Let these herbs introduce you to the world of plant remedies, and you'll develop a deep well of experience to draw from when you meet other herbs in the future.

Angelica Angelica archangelica

Qualities: warming, drying, tonifying

Taste: bitter, pungent, aromatic

Family: Apiaceae

Medicinal parts: root, seed, stems

Actions: alterative, antimicrobial, aromatic, bitter, carminative, circulatory stimulant, diaphoretic, diffusive, emmenagogue, expectorant, grounding, nervine

Common Preparations

Angelica roots can be decocted, and both the roots and the seeds can be prepared as infusions, tinctures, or elixirs. The stems can be candied or cooked and eaten.

Ideal for Addressing

- ADD/ADHD
- Bloating
- BPH/prostatitis
- Chest cold/bronchitis/pneumonia
- Constipation
- Cough
- Fatigue
- Fever
- PMS
- Seasonal depression
- Varicose veins and hemorrhoids

Effective Applications

Angelica is a strongly grounding plant, acting to calm and support the nervous system. This makes angelica particularly helpful for issues like ADD and ADHD, anxiety, and overstimulation. Angelica's grounding effects, combined with its circulatory stimulant action, are also helpful in cases of cyclic depression, such as seasonal depression or PMS.

That warming, blood-moving action is also effective on a physical level for issues from bloating to edema to constipation: Angelica gets things moving! This makes angelica very handy in any formula targeting stagnation and sluggishness in the body.

Angelica is one of the few warming digestive bitters—important because cold, sluggish digestion is so common in our culture. In addition to improving digestion by warming the digestive tract, angelica can help release stress, which makes it easier to digest food. A dropperful of angelica tincture before a meal is an easy way to improve digestion and release stress—all in one.

Angelica's expectorant action is particularly helpful for wet, phlegmy coughs. Decoct the roots with a heavy lid to retain the aromatic, volatile oils. When you ladle out a cup, breathe in the steam as it cools to increase angelica's antimicrobial action in the respiratory tract.

Angelica blends particularly well with ashwagandha and decaf coffee for a delicious decoction. Although there's no caffeine, angelica makes it easier to manage stress and keep going strong, all day long.

Recommended Dosage

Angelica is an herb commonly used as food and can be consumed safely in food-like quantities. For respiratory ailments, 3 to 4 cups of tea a day, sipped slowly, will be effective. For improving digestion, 1 to 2 droppersful of tincture before each meal or snack is sufficient. For bloating, a cup of tea as needed. For circulatory support, fatigue, and other longer-term issues, plan to incorporate angelica into your life at least 3 times a day as tea or tincture, alone or in formula.

Important Considerations

Because angelica stimulates circulation and is particularly influential on the reproductive system, it can improve blood flow in individuals with sluggish menstruation. For those prone to heavy periods, though, angelica is best avoided in the week before menstruation.

Do not take angelica in high doses if you take pharmaceutical blood thinners.

Angelica archangelica is not the same plant as Chinese angelica (*A. sinensis*), often referred to as dong quai or dang gui.

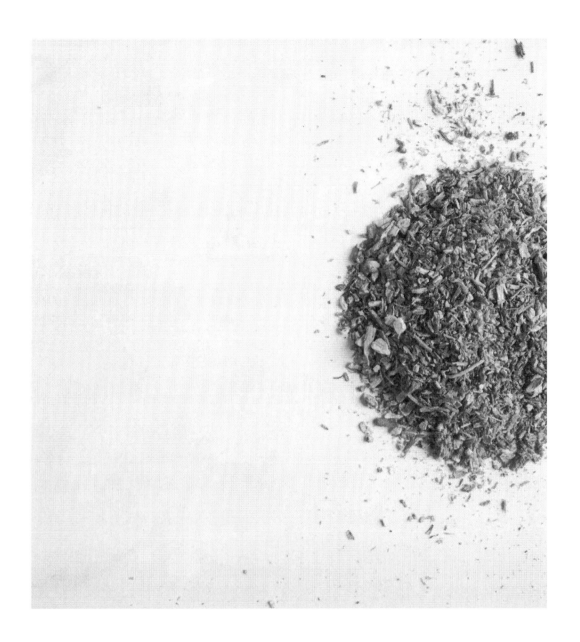

Ashwagandha Withania somnifera

Qualities: warming, drying, relaxant
Taste: bitter, sweet, pungent
Family: Solanaceae
Medicinal parts: root
Actions: adaptogen, alterative, antispasmodic, cardiac tonic, immunomodulator, nervous trophorestorative

Common Preparations

Ashwagandha root can be decocted, tinctured, powdered, or prepared as an elixir.

Ideal for Addressing

* ADD/ADHD
* Depression
* Fatigue
* Hypothyroidism
* Insomnia
* Menopause/andropause
* Menstrual cycle irregularities
* PMS
* Seasonal depression
* Stress

Effective Applications

Ashwagandha is one of the *adaptogenic* herbs that help the body cope with stress more easily. Most of this action comes by improving the function of the adrenal glands and the rest of the endocrine system, which is responsible for orchestrating the entire symphony of the body's functions. Ashwagandha is a great herb to "tune-up" the whole system, especially during times of stress and heavy workloads.

Ashwagandha helps the body stick to its circadian rhythm, so it's easier to fall asleep at night and stay active and wakeful during the day. As a result, it can be particularly helpful for addressing "out of cycle" situations, like insomnia or seasonal depression. Because ashwagandha supports the "rest and digest" functions of the body and can soothe an overstimulated nervous system, it's also great for relieving anxiety and feelings of overwhelm.

Ashwagandha might be translated as "strength of a thousand horses," but its action is quite a bit more gentle and foundational than the image conjured up by the translation! Unlike more stimulating herbs, such as ginseng or eleuthero, ashwagandha is a slow, restorative builder. There's no big rush of energy, which means there's no corresponding crash of energy running out. Instead, each day you have a little more resilience than the day before—until, after a while, you feel like your old self again! Ashwagandha is particularly appropriate in cases of extended exhaustion, depletion, and deficiency.

Recommended Dosage

Ashwagandha is not a particularly delicious herb, but it can be blended in many ways that cover the taste. Chai spices, such as ginger, cardamom, and cinnamon, are strong, familiar flavors that can do the trick; so is coffee. Drink 1 to 4 cups of these blends daily. Ashwagandha can also be taken as tincture (1 to 8 droppersful per day), or as a honey powder paste (1 to 3 tablespoons per day). When getting to sleep and staying asleep is an issue, pulse dosing before bed is effective: Take 3 droppersful of tincture 1 hour before bedtime, the same amount half an hour before bedtime, and again right at bedtime. With consistent use over 1 week to 1 month, you'll see drastic changes in your sleep quality. Ashwagandha works best with consistent, long-term use.

Important Considerations

Ashwagandha is a nightshade plant, and may need to be avoided by people with allergies to tomatoes, potatoes, eggplant, etc.

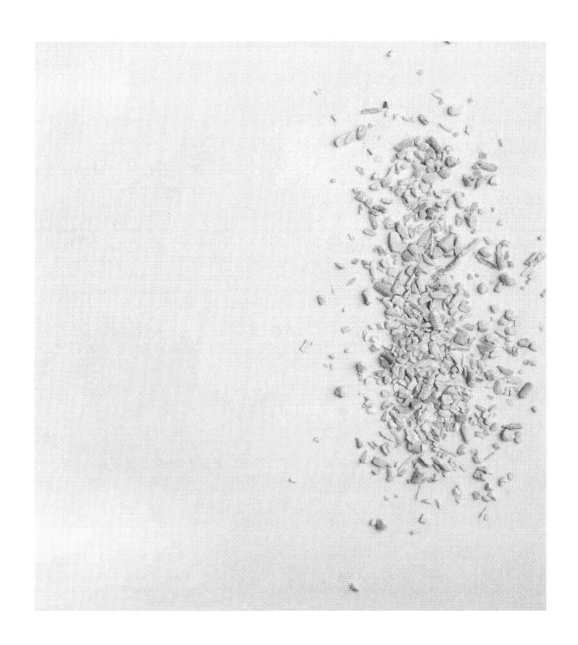

<u>Betony</u> Stachys officinalis (S. betonica, Betonica off.)

Qualities: neutral, drying, relaxant
Taste: mildly bitter, aromatic, slightly sweet
Family: Lamiaceae
Medicinal parts: leaves and flowers
Actions: anxiolytic, antispasmodic, diaphoretic, diffusive, grounding, hepatic, mildly astringent, nervine

Common Preparations

The leaves and flowers of betony can be infused as tea or prepared as a tincture or elixir.

Ideal for Addressing

* ADD/ADHD
* Anxiety
* Depression
* Headache
* Heart palpitations
* Menstrual cycle irregularities
* PMS
* Stress

Effective Applications

One of the best herbs for all kinds of head ailments, betony is a top choice for many types of headaches: tension headaches, hormonal or menstrual headaches, migraines, cluster headaches, and chronic headaches. Betony releases tension in constricted muscles, especially in the neck and head. It's a traditional remedy for seizure disorders and spastic conditions characterized by tremors and shaking, as well as concussion.

Betony is helpful for people who easily get lost in their thoughts and need help staying grounded and connected to their body. It's especially appropriate for people experiencing dissociation, or a disconnect between their mind and body, and people who work heavily with machines and computers, as it can bring the focus out of the cerebral head-space and back into the present moment.

Because betony strengthens the mind-body connection, it is beneficial for people suffering from depression and adolescents going through puberty—two populations that often struggle with difficult thoughts and emotions. Add that to the grounding, antispasmodic, and diffusive actions and you have an ideal remedy for issues such as heart palpitations, stress, anxiety, and ADD/ADHD.

Recommended Dosage

Betony is mild enough in flavor to drink on its own as a tea, but it lends itself beautifully to formulation. Tulsi, chamomile, rose, catnip, and linden pair well with betony, both in flavor and effect. For headache, a cup of betony tea, as needed, may be sufficient. For long-term support with issues such as dissociative disorders, anxiety, and post-concussive stresses, 2 to 4 cups of betony daily, alone or in formula, over several weeks or months, is more appropriate.

Important Considerations

Two different plants are known as betony in the United States: *Stachys officinalis* and *Pedicularis spp.* We are referring to *Stachys off.*, though *Pedicularis* has some of the same effects.

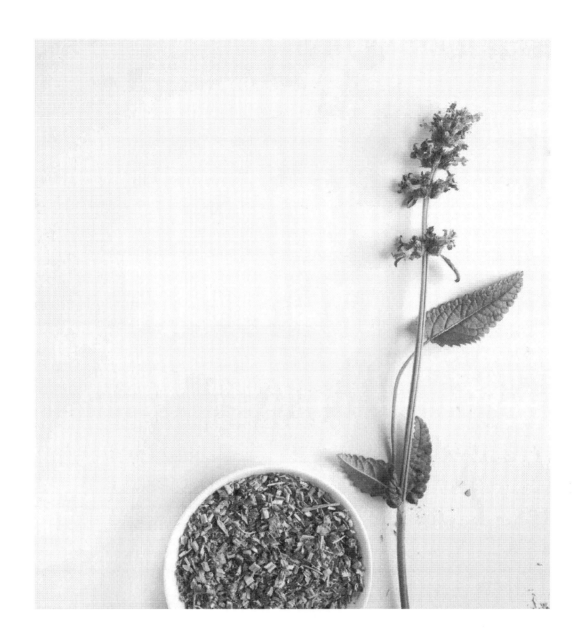

Calendula Calendula officinalis

Qualities: warming, drying, tonifying
Taste: bitter, pungent, salty, sweet
Family: Asteraceae
Medicinal parts: flowers
Actions: alterative, antifungal, antimicrobial, diaphoretic, lymphatic, vulnerary

Common Preparations

The calendula flower head can be infused for a tea or a compress or prepared as a tincture, elixir, or salve.

Ideal for Addressing

- Abscess and gingivitis
- Acne
- Allergies
- Athlete's foot/fungal skin infections
- Bloating
- BPH/prostatitis
- Breast fibroids and cysts
- Burns and sunburn
- Detox
- Eczema and dermatitis
- Edema
- Endometriosis
- Food sensitivities
- Gingivitis

- IBS/IBD/ulcerative colitis
- Indigestion/dyspepsia
- Inflammation
- Leaky gut
- Menopause/andropause
- PMS
- Rash
- Receding gums
- Seasonal depression
- Stomach ulcer/gastritis
- Varicose veins and hemorrhoids
- Wounds
- Yeast infection

Effective Applications

Many digestive system ailments share a similar symptom triangle: irritation and inflammation in the gastrointestinal tract, impaired digestive and liver function, and a lymphatic response such as bloating. Calendula is effective for all three! Tea is the most effective way to work with calendula for digestive ailments.

Calendula's liver-stimulating action makes it helpful for issues where hormones play a role, such as endometriosis and PMS symptoms. The lymphatic action is also supportive for fibroids and cysts, inflammatory issues, many types of rashes, varicose veins—anything that has a component of lymphatic stagnancy. With those actions together, calendula is well suited for a wide variety of conditions that involve water retention, such as intestinal bloating, edema, and BPH. Because ailments on these lists often occur together, calendula gets you two (or more) treatments in one!

The digestive tract cells are the same type of cells that make up skin, which is why calendula is fantastic for healing wounds and irritation in both areas. It's important to get the herb directly in contact with the wound, which means tea for digestive tract use, and a compress, soak, or salve for skin issues.

Recommended Dosage

Calendula is safe to work with in food-like doses. For chronic internal issues, we recommend a quart of tea daily, either on its own or as part of a formula. For topical issues, application of calendula by compress, soak, or salve multiple times a day is appropriate until the issue resolves. Calendula is also a sunny, friendly plant and can be added to any formula just to bring in that brightness!

Important Considerations

Calendula is a very safe plant and is appropriate even for newborns and elders.

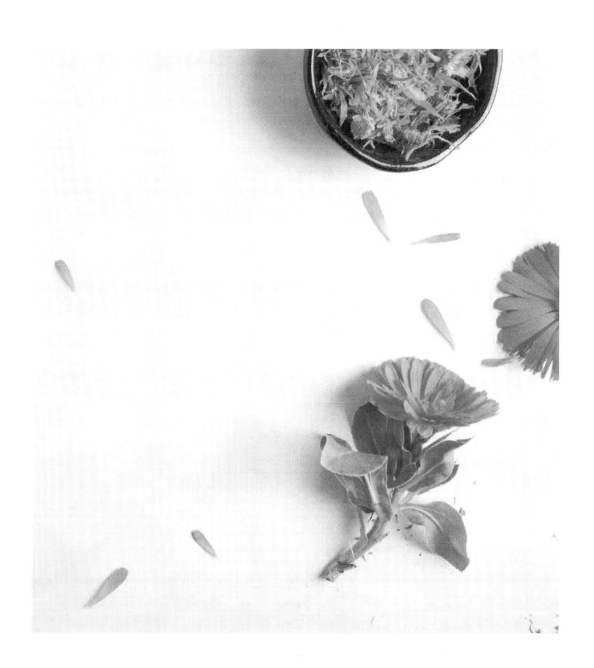

Catnip_Nepeta cataria

Qualities: warming, drying, relaxant
Taste: pungent, aromatic, acrid
Family: Lamiaceae
Medicinal parts: leaves and flowers
Actions: antispasmodic, anxiolytic, aromatic, carminative, diaphoretic, hepatic, nervine, sedative

Common Preparations

Catnip leaves and flowers can be infused as a tea or prepared as a tincture or elixir.

Ideal for Addressing

* ADD/ADHD
* Anxiety
* Fever
* Food sensitivities
* Heartburn/reflux/gastroesophageal reflux disease (GERD)
* IBS/IBD/ulcerative colitis
* Indigestion/dyspepsia
* Leaky gut
* Nausea

Effective Applications

Catnip's relaxant and digestive actions make this a very effective plant for anxiety or nervousness, especially when poor digestive function is also involved. Catnip is particularly indicated when this nervous energy or upset has an upward-moving direction, as in heartburn and "butterflies in the stomach." For headaches caused by poor or incomplete digestion, catnip is an effective remedy, especially when combined with another warming or carminative herb like sage or fennel.

Somewhat sedative, catnip can be helpful for panic and anxiety in adults and children. A soothing herb, catnip is a nice nervine to take before bedtime, either alone or added to a sedative formula for times when falling asleep is difficult. Tea, tincture, or elixir all work well to support sleep.

As a relaxing diaphoretic, catnip relaxes muscles to allow a fever's heat to escape the body. Catnip is commonly included in formulas to break a high or long-lasting fever. This same action can be applied emotionally, as well: When emotions are running hot and you can't let go of them, try catnip!

Ryn would like to remind you: Catnip is actually good for cats! Felines aren't very interested in most plants, but catnip gets their attention because its aromatic constituents are similar to their pheromones. Observe closely when you give catnip to your cats: After they run around a bit, you'll notice they settle in and purr contentedly. When you could use a good purr yourself, think of catnip.

Recommended Dosage

One cup of catnip tea is effective for relief in the moment, but for long-term issues, it's a great idea to have catnip regularly. Three to 4 cups daily, alone or in formula, is ideal. Tincture and elixir are safe to use regularly and as needed in doses of 1 to 8 droppersful.

Important Considerations

Catnip is a safe herb for children, although it is more strongly sedating for them than it is for adults.

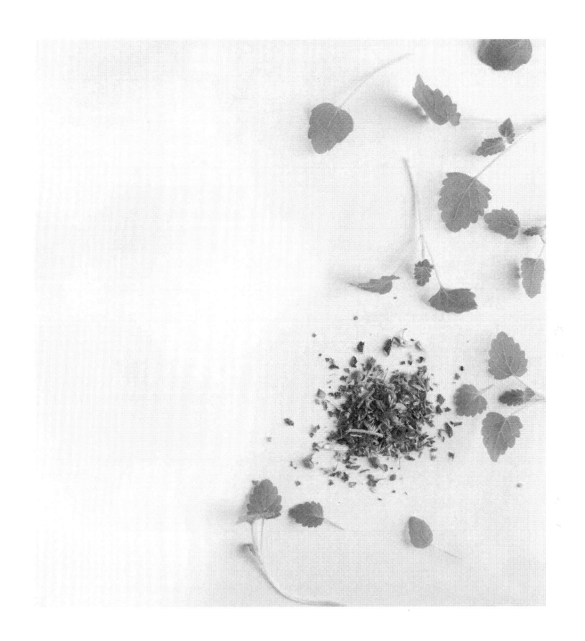

Chamomile Matricaria recutita

Qualities: warming, neutral, relaxant

Taste: aromatic, bitter, sweet **Family:** Asteraceae

Medicinal parts: flowers

Actions: antimicrobial, antispasmodic, anxiolytic, aromatic, carminative, sedative, soothing nervine, stomach tonic, vulnerary

Common Preparations

Chamomile flowers can be infused as tea or a compress or prepared as a tincture, elixir, or salve.

Ideal for Addressing

* Abscess
* Acne
* ADD/ADHD
* Anxiety
* Depression
* Eczema and dermatitis
* Food sensitivities
* Headache
* Heart palpitations
* IBS/IBD/ulcerative colitis
* Indigestion/dyspepsia
* Insomnia
* Leaky gut
* Menstrual cycle irregularities

- Pain management
- Plantar fasciitis
- Receding gums
- Stress
- Wounds

Effective Applications

Perhaps because it is considered gentle, or perhaps because it is a ubiquitous tea, chamomile is often undervalued in our culture. Yet in other cultures, chamomile is prized for its powerful wound-healing abilities. For serious wounds, it's probably better to visit the emergency room, but for everyday cuts and scrapes, you can rely on a wash or a soak with strong chamomile tea to aid a speedy recovery.

Chamomile is the ideal choice for people who run cold and damp physically, but have type A personalities. There's no single better plant for helping relax and unwind before bed—or anytime! Have tea or elixir by itself, or blend with ginger, betony, and/or elderflower for a tremendously effective relaxant. Chamomile is also excellent for headaches caused by mental tension.

The antispasmodic action of chamomile is also very potent, but for this effect you'll need a strong cup of tea. If you have teabags, put three or four in your cup; if you have loose leaf, use 1 tablespoon per cup. Either way, cover and steep it long enough to become noticeably bitter. The flavor may not be as pleasant as a lighter, shorter steep, but the results are absolutely worth it. This is effective for menstrual cramps, intestinal cramping, headaches, and general muscle tension.

Recommended Dosage

Chamomile can be taken freely as needed. Consider a cup of chamomile tea with ginger in the evening to help relax, especially when there is tension or digestive distress. For wound care or other topical applications, apply as a compress, soak, or steam multiple times a day. Three to 4 cups of chamomile daily, alone or in formula, are very helpful for chronic digestive issues.

Important Considerations

Chamomile is a very safe herb that is particularly nice for children (and dogs, too!). Occasionally, people have hay fever-like allergies to chamomile and other daisy family (Asteraceae) plants.

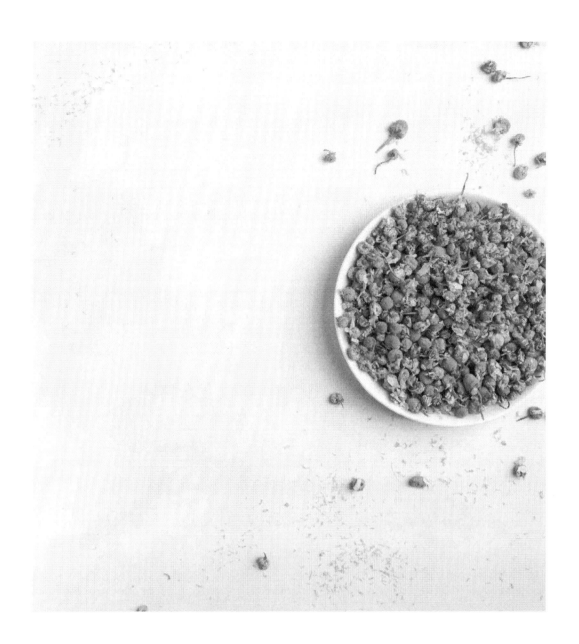

Cinnamon Cinnamomum cassia

Qualities: warming, moistening, tonifying

Taste: pungent, sweet, astringent **Family:**
Lauraceae

Medicinal parts: inner bark

Actions: antimicrobial, aromatic, astringent, demulcent, diffusive, hypoglycemic, mild circulatory stimulant, relaxant

Common Preparations

Cinnamon can be prepared as a hot or cold infusion or a decoction. Cinnamon essential oil can be added to salves. Cinnamon can also be added to food.

Ideal for Addressing

* Athlete's foot/fungal skin infections
* Bloating
* Fever
* Hypoglycemia
* Indigestion/dyspepsia
* PCOS
* Sore throat and respiratory ailments

Effective Applications

Both warming *and* moistening when prepared in water, cinnamon is excellent for cold, dry conditions, such as sluggish digestion and constipation. That warm, moist quality is also very helpful for dry, sore throats and coughs. Cinnamon can be taken on its own as tea or added to other formulas for its own actions and to improve the flavor of less-tasty herbs. To get the full range of warmth and moistening action, first prepare hot cinnamon tea, then let sit for a few hours after it has cooled: The moistening constituents are only soluble in cool water. Strain the tea before reheating gently to retain all the moistening action, and enjoy warm.

Cinnamon is a very potent antifungal agent. Cinnamon powder can be regularly applied directly to the affected area when that is convenient (for example, as a foot powder for athlete's foot) or applied as a salve. Cinnamon essential oil can be added to salves made with calendula—the two plants together form a powerful pair.

Cinnamon is an effective ally for insulin resistance and pre-diabetes, as well as symptoms arising from those conditions, such as polycystic ovary syndrome (PCOS). In a 2003 study published in *Diabetes Care*, researchers found that 1 gram (about ½ teaspoon) of cinnamon daily was enough to reduce blood glucose levels significantly, as well as cholesterol and triglyceride levels in people with type 2 diabetes. Those are very encouraging results, especially for people not yet medicated and working to avoid worsening symptoms. It is important to test glucose levels daily and communicate with your doctor if you take medication for diabetes.

Recommended Dosage

Cinnamon is very safe in cooking and is often included in sweet recipes or heavier recipes where its warming action can assist in digestion. For sore throat, cinnamon tea can be taken as needed throughout the day. For fungal infections, cinnamon preparations can be applied several times a day as needed—though it is not recommended to apply essential oils directly to the skin without diluting them first.

Important Considerations

Due to cinnamon's effect on blood glucose, people taking Glucophage (metformin) or using insulin injections need to monitor their glucose levels when taking cinnamon in doses larger than culinary amounts, as blood sugar levels can change quickly. In large doses, cinnamon has a blood-thinning effect, and high amounts of cinnamon (greater than 6 grams per day) should be avoided if you take blood-thinning pharmaceuticals.

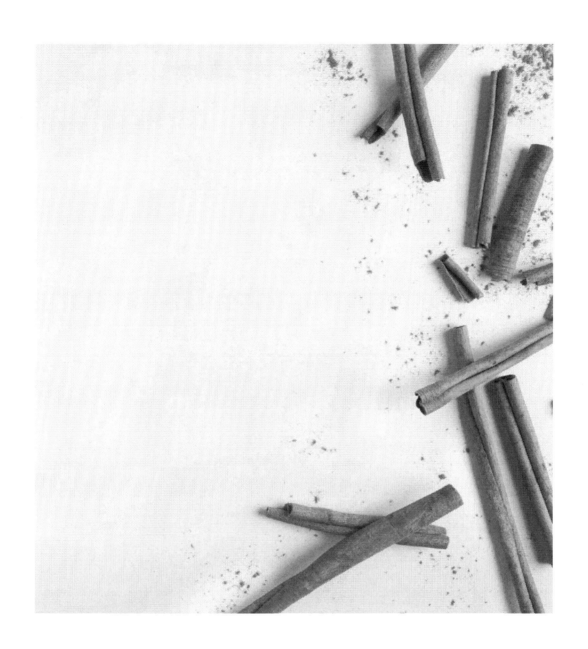

Dandelion Taraxacum officinale

Qualities: cooling, drying, tonifying
Taste: bitter, earthy, sweet, salty
Family: Asteraceae
Medicinal parts: root, leaves, flowers
Actions: leaves—alterative, antilithic, diuretic, drying, nutritive; root—antilithic cholagogue, mild laxative, sialagogue; flowers—exhilarant

Common Preparations

Dandelion leaves can be infused for tea: A long infusion (4 to 8 hours) releases the most mineral content. Dandelion leaves can also be tinctured in vinegar or eaten as food. Dandelion roots can be decocted as tea or prepared as tincture. Dandelion flowers can be prepared as a honey infusion, tincture, or elixir.

Ideal for Addressing

* Acne
* Constipation
* Detox
* Dry mouth
* Eczema
* Endometriosis
* Gout
* Kidney stones
* Menstrual cycle irregularities
* PCOS
* PMS
* Rash

- Varicose veins and hemorrhoids

Effective Applications

Dandelion flowers can be infused into honey or tinctured for an emotionally uplifting action.

Dandelion roots and leaves are applicable at different times: Dandelion roots act more strongly on the liver and digestive system, and their stimulating effect on the liver improves the body's ability to digest food and detox. This has fairly far-reaching effects, from improving acne, eczema, and rashes to reducing constipation. The liver's detox functions are responsible for breaking down excess hormones in the body, which means the root can even be an effective helper for those with hormonal conditions such as PCOS and PMS.

Dandelion roots also contain inulin, a *prebiotic* fiber that feeds probiotic gut flora. Inulin is most available in a decoction, so blend dandelion roots with chai spices or decaf coffee for a daily morning blend to support digestion.

Dandelion leaves act more strongly on the kidneys, have higher mineral content, and are more astringent. The leaf's high mineral content supports healthy kidney function. Both the improvements in kidney function and the minerals themselves can drastically reduce PMS symptoms and endometriosis, and help create a more regular menstrual cycle. The leaf is also very helpful for treating gout and protecting against kidney stones, and its astringent action helps drain extra fluid from the body, as in edema and water retention. This diuretic action can also reduce high blood pressure and is best attained by taking daily doses of long-infused dandelion leaf tea. That astringency is also supportive for varicose veins and hemorrhoids, especially when combined with topical preparations.

Recommended Dosage

Dandelion is a "food herb," and is coming back into fashion in salads and other dishes. Eating dandelion leaves is a great way to receive the benefits of this plant! Dandelion leaf's nourishing infusion is most supportive when taken over time; drink 2 to 3 cups daily, either alone or as part of a formula.

Dandelion roots are also traditionally eaten as food, and their benefits are similarly best seen when they become a consistent part of your daily routine. Take root tincture in doses of 1 to 4 droppersful 3 times per day, or drink 2 to 4 cups of decoction, alone or in a formula.

Important Considerations

Dandelion leaf should be paired with moistening herbs such as linden or licorice for people with very dry constitutions. *Dandelion leaves may not be suitable for people taking blood thinners or pharmaceutical diuretics.*

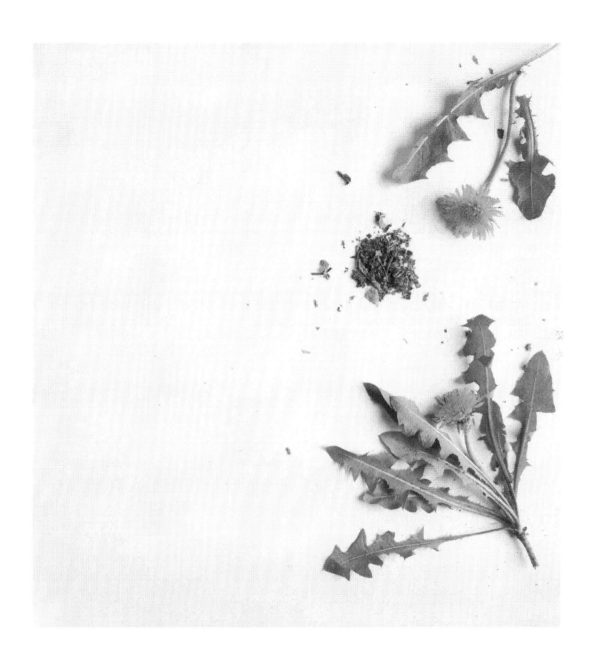

<u>Elder</u> Sambucus nigra, S. canadensis

Qualities: cooling, drying, relaxant
Taste: sweet, slightly oily, astringent
Family: Adoxaceae
Medicinal parts: berries and flowers
Actions: alterative, antimicrobial, antitussive, antiviral, astringent, diaphoretic, diuretic, exhilarant, immune stimulant, nutritive, relaxant, respiratory antispasmodic

Common Preparations

Both elderflowers and elderberries can be prepared as tea, tincture, elixir, syrup, and honey infusion. Elderflowers are also made into liqueurs, sold commercially.

Ideal for Addressing

* Anxiety
* Bronchitis/chest cold/pneumonia
* Cold and flu
* Depression
* Fever
* Immune support
* PMS
* Stress

Effective Applications

Today, elder may be best known for its ability to prevent viruses from replicating, especially influenza viruses, making it much easier for the immune system to fight these pathogens. This decreases the severity and length of the illness. Elder also has a stimulating effect on immune function. These actions are strongest in the berries but are also present in the flowers. Elderberries can even help preserve immune function as we age, due to their high antioxidant content.

Elderflowers are a relaxing diaphoretic, meaning they assist in "sweating out" a fever. Elder is especially helpful when fever and chills alternate. A hot cup of tea is the best preparation for this result. This diaphoretic action can also work emotionally, helping release intense emotions or worry and allowing the mind to relax.

Katja particularly loves a blend of elderflower, chamomile, and linden to help relax her "type A" personality at the end of the day. This can be made into a tasty tea with equal parts of each herb. Served with a spoonful of honey, it is a great way to transition from work to home.

Recommended Dosage

Elderberries can be eaten as jam or jelly, or baked into other foods. For colds and flu, 1 tablespoon of syrup 3 to 4 times daily at the first sign of symptoms is ideal; this can be continued until you recover. Elderflowers can be taken freely as hot tea for fever or stress management or as a tincture or elixir for releasing feelings of stress.

Unlike some immune-stimulating herbs, elder is typically well tolerated in individuals with autoimmune conditions.

Important Considerations

Large amounts of fresh elderberries have a laxative effect. Cook elderberries for food use.

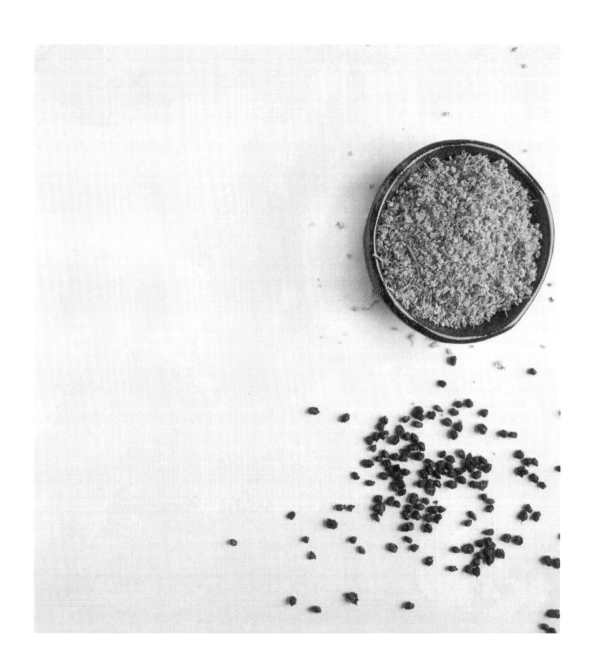

Elecampane Inula helenium

Qualities: warming, drying, tonifying
Taste: pungent, bitter
Family: Asteraceae
Medicinal parts: root
Actions: antimicrobial, bitter, diaphoretic, emmenagogue, expectorant, nervous system tonic, nutritive, respiratory stimulant

Common Preparations

Elecampane roots are best decocted for tea, although they can be infused for a lighter effect. They can also be prepared as a tincture.

Ideal for Addressing

* Asthma
* Bronchitis/chest cold/pneumonia
* Cough
* Immune support
* Indigestion and dyspepsia

Effective Applications

Elecampane is particularly suited to treat infections of the respiratory tract, especially those that come with thick, heavy mucus. Its antimicrobial effect kills bacteria, while the stimulating and expectorating actions help bring up the stuck, thick mucus that accumulates at the bottom of the lungs, which can otherwise be very difficult to get rid of.

Elecampane is one of the most strongly antiseptic plants in our *materia medica* (collection of medicinal plants). Particularly effective for bacterial infections, elecampane has been successful against bronchitis, pneumonia, tuberculosis, and MRSA, in part due to its biofilm-disrupting action, which makes it more difficult for pathogens to defend themselves against our immune systems.

Elecampane contains a high percentage of inulin, a prebiotic fiber that is a preferred food for healthy gut bacteria. Elecampane is also a warming, digestive bitter and a liver stimulant. These functions work together to help fight dysbiosis in the gut and can speed recovery from food-borne infection.

Recommended Dosage

Elecampane's flavor might be best described as "peppery mud," but it is so effective it's worth putting up with. Instead of drinking an entire cup of decoction, take 1 or 2 tablespoons every hour, from the first sign of respiratory infection until the illness clears. Alternatively, blending elecampane with other pungent respiratory herbs, such as ginger, angelica, and cinnamon, can help mask its flavor.

Elecampane's inulin content will sink to the bottom of the brew: If you want to work with the inulin, give the decoction a good stir before ladling out a cup. Inulin is not well extracted by alcohol, so a decoction is the preferred method for this application.

Important Considerations

People with allergies to members of the daisy plant family (Asteraceae) may be allergic to elecampane. This is uncommon, in our experience.

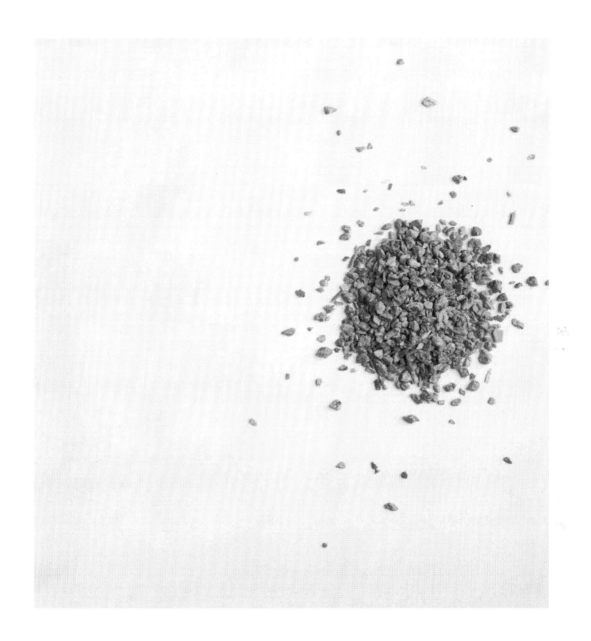

Fennel Foeniculum vulgare

Qualities: warming, moistening, relaxant
Taste: aromatic, pungent, sweet
Family: Apiaceae
Medicinal parts: seed
Actions: antiemetic, antispasmodic, aromatic, carminative, cholagogue, diuretic, galactagogue, sialagogue

Common Preparations

Fennel seeds can be eaten as they are, added to food, infused for tea, or tinctured.

Ideal for Addressing

* Asthma
* Bloating
* Food sensitivities
* IBS/IBD/ulcerative colitis
* Indigestion/dyspepsia
* Leaky gut
* PMS

Effective Applications

A warming herb that improves digestion and liver function, fennel is particularly suited to counteract the cold, stagnant conditions we see so commonly in our population today. Fennel can help relieve gas and bloating in adults and children, and colic in babies. Fennel can be added directly to foods likely to cause gas or bloating or taken as tea after the meal. For babies, a little bit of fennel tea on a spoon or given by dropper can be quite effective.

Fennel is antispasmodic, making it a helpful remedy for intestinal cramping, whether it's a bout of indigestion or part of something chronic, such as IBS. The antispasmodic action is also effective for soothing menstrual cramping and relieving the constriction and spasms of asthma.

We particularly like to include fennel in our <u>Gut-Heal Tea</u>, which is a universal blend that can apply to a wide variety of digestive complaints, both chronic and acute.

Recommended Dosage

Fennel is common in cooking for the same reasons it can be helpful as an herbal preparation: It improves digestion! You may already include fennel in recipes with fattier cuts of meat or sausage, where it stimulates digestion to improve the body's ability to digest that fat. Fennel is safe to eat as food, and infusions of fennel can be taken as often as desired.

Important Considerations

Fennel is very safe for humans of all ages.

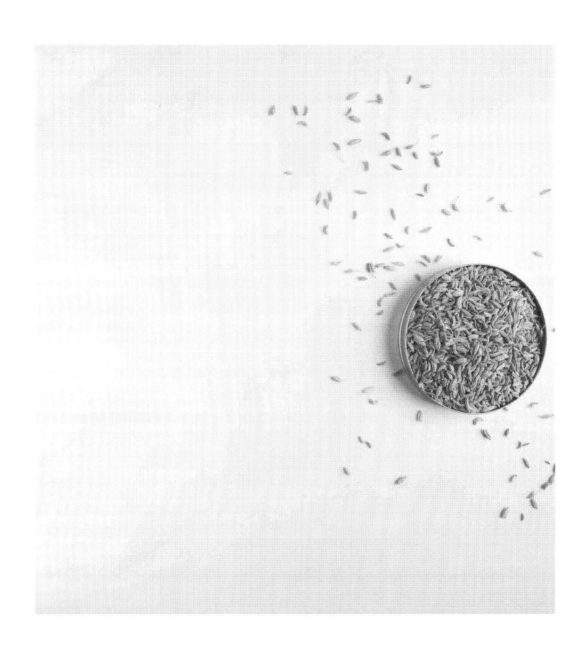

Garlic Allium sativum

Qualities: warming, drying, tonifying
Taste: pungent, aromatic, oily, slightly sweet
Family: Amaryllidaceae
Medicinal parts: bulb
Actions: alterative, antifungal, anti-inflammatory, antimicrobial, aromatic, carminative, circulatory stimulant, diffusive, hepatic stimulant, hypotensive, rubefacient

Common Preparations

Garlic can be eaten in food, prepared by pickling in vinegar and honey, made into tea, added to broth, or infused into oil. It can also be prepared in water or vinegar for topical applications or as a steam.

Ideal for Addressing

- Athlete's foot/fungal skin infections
- Bronchitis/chest cold/pneumonia
- Cholesterol management
- Cold and flu
- Dysbiosis
- Ear infection/earache
- Immune support
- Sinusitis/stuffy nose

Effective Applications

Garlic is a vital plant for managing respiratory tract infections, including cold, flu, pneumonia, bronchitis, tonsillitis, strep throat, and sinus infections. This is because some of the most antimicrobial aspects of garlic you've ingested exit the body through the lungs as you exhale—that's how you get garlic breath. On the way out, they directly destroy fungi and bacteria while stimulating an immune response against viruses in the mucous membranes. This makes garlic a remedy specific to microbial infections of the lungs.

These antimicrobial agents function anywhere they can reach, so topical application of garlic—to a wound on the skin, in the digestive tract, or at the site of other infections—will also be antibacterial and antifungal. However, raw garlic can also cause damage to skin and digestive tract tissue, so it's important to buffer garlic's heating action with oil when applying it to the skin and to be conscious of your body's reaction when consuming raw garlic. If raw garlic is too intense, consider "pickling" it—combine peeled garlic cloves in a jar with half apple cider vinegar and half honey and let soak for a month. Garlic pickles retain all the benefits but are gentler on the digestive system.

By improving the quality of the blood and stimulating circulation while lowering blood pressure, garlic can have beneficial effects on the cardiovascular system. Plus, garlic is packed with antioxidants, which help lower cholesterol levels.

Because garlic's aromatic oils are exhaled through your lungs, you can have "garlic breath" even if you didn't actually eat any garlic. Try applying garlic to your feet, either with an application of infused oil or a soak in garlic tea or vinegar. Within 5 to 10 minutes, you'll be breathing garlic!

Garlic can be taken as tea for respiratory infections, or added to broth, and it pairs well with thyme for this purpose. Garlic and thyme tea is Ryn's first line of attack when he notices a cold or the flu coming on.

Recommended Dosage

Garlic is safe to consume in food amounts daily. Raw garlic can irritate the stomach and skin, but garlic preparations do not typically present this problem. Be attentive; if the feeling is too hot, take a break. Garlic can be taken medicinally in many forms—simply adding it to food is a great way to make garlic's benefits a regular part of your life. A garlic steam (see Sinus-Clearing Steam) is an intense experience, but tremendously effective for beating colds and flu. Garlic infused into vinegar is a fantastic way to apply the fungus-fighting action directly to the affected area—multiple times a day is ideal.

Important Considerations

Garlic can be very irritating to skin and the digestive tract when applied raw. Garlic has a strong blood-thinning effect. This can be problematic for individuals taking blood-thinning pharmaceuticals; *check with your doctor before adding garlic to your regimen if you take one of those drugs.* Occasionally, people do have allergies to garlic.

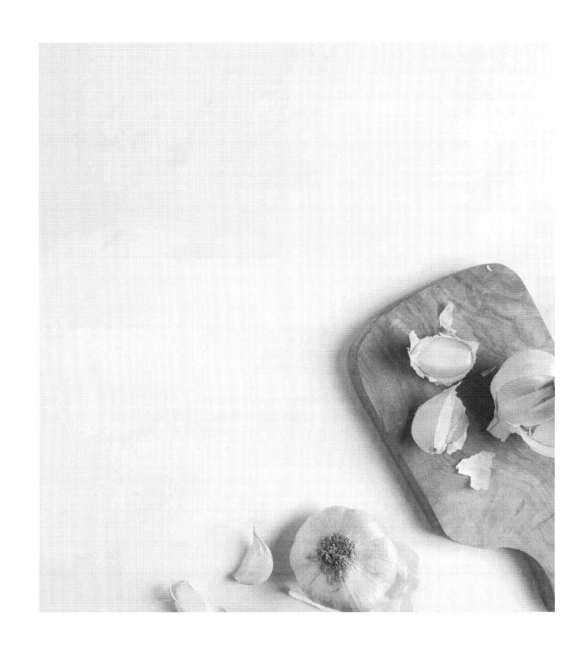

Ginger Zingiber officinale

Qualities: warming, drying, relaxant
Taste: pungent, aromatic
Family: Zingiberaceae
Medicinal parts: rhizome (root)
Actions: anodyne, antiemetic, anti-inflammatory, antispasmodic, aromatic, carminative, diaphoretic, diffusive, emmenagogue, relaxant, rubefacient, sialagogue, stimulant, stomach tonic

Common Preparations

Ginger can be added to food, made as tea, and even candied for medicinal use. Tincture of ginger can be used internally and topically or blended into an elixir for a tasty remedy.

Ideal for Addressing

* Arthritis
* Back pain
* Bloating and intestinal cramping
* BPH/prostatitis
* Bronchitis/chest cold/pneumonia
* Constipation
* Cough
* Dry mouth
* Endometriosis
* Fever
* Headache
* Heart palpitations
* IBS/IBD/ulcerative colitis

- Inflammation
- Joint pain
- Menstrual cycle irregularities
- Muscle soreness/post-workout recovery
- Nausea
- Pain management
- Plantar fasciitis
- PMS
- Seasonal depression
- Sprains and strains
- Varicose veins and hemorrhoids

Effective Applications

Ginger has a particularly effective combination of actions—especially its warming antispasmodic and anti-inflammatory actions—that make it appropriate for a wide variety of ailments.

Ginger's warming quality can stimulate digestion, resolving slow and sluggish issues such as bloating and constipation. Combined with ginger's antispasmodic actions, the result is a very effective treatment for gut cramping—whether from IBS, PMS, or some food that didn't agree with you. This warming, relaxant action also makes ginger ideal for headaches and backaches resulting from tension, or those that come along with digestive or menstrual problems.

Ginger can also stimulate circulation, improving blood flow throughout the body. Along with its anti-inflammatory action, this makes ginger very effective for treating cardiovascular problems and issues that result from systemic inflammation (such as rheumatoid arthritis). This also encourages healthy menstrual flow.

Ryn likes powdered ginger in a honey powder paste—1 or 2 tablespoons, spread on toast or mixed into hot cereal, really warms the belly on a cold winter's morning.

Ginger is very effective against all forms of nausea, including those induced by food poisoning, medications (including chemotherapy), morning sickness, and motion sickness.

A warming diaphoretic, ginger encourages a healthy fever in response to infection.

All these actions combine to help ginger effectively counter many types of depression: The circulatory stimulant action helps the body feel more alive, and the antispasmodic action can help release anxiety or other stressors contributing to the problem. As researchers continue to investigate the connection between inflammation and depression, we will likely see more ways ginger can support people experiencing depression.

Recommended Dosage

Ginger is common in recipes, and food is a great way to get ginger into your life. Ginger can also be taken in tea as needed for headaches, cramps, and digestive problems or daily for chronic and inflammatory issues—3 to 4 cups daily is a good target. Tincture of ginger works well in doses as small as a few drops, though 4 or more droppersful may be taken at once for some purposes. Ginger blends well with many herbs and can enhance the unappealing flavor of some herbs. Ginger can also be applied topically, as needed, in a tincture or liniment (see here and here).

Important Considerations

Ginger has a blood-thinning effect; *if you take blood-thinning medications, consult your doctor.* Ginger's emmenagogic action may increase the menstrual flow of those with already heavy cycles.

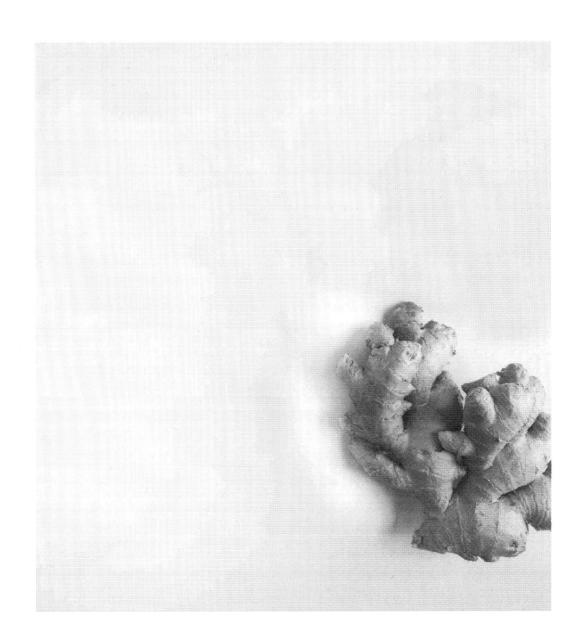

Goldenrod Solidago spp.

Qualities: warming, drying, tonifying

Taste: aromatic, bitter, astringent

Family: Asteraceae

Medicinal parts: leaves and flowers

Actions: analgesic, anticatarrhal, anti-inflammatory, antilithic, antispasmodic, aromatic, astringent, carminative, diuretic, urinary antiseptic, vulnerary

Common Preparations

Goldenrod can be prepared as tea or tincture or infused into oil to make a salve.

Ideal for Addressing

- Abscess and gingivitis
- Allergies
- Anxiety
- Back pain
- Depression
- Detox
- Endometriosis
- Gingivitis
- Gout
- Heartburn/reflux/GERD
- Insomnia
- Kidney stones
- Menstrual cycle irregularities
- Muscle soreness/post-workout recovery

- PMS
- Receding gums
- Seasonal depression
- Sore throat
- Stomach ulcer/gastritis
- Stress
- Urinary tract infection (UTI)
- Varicose veins and hemorrhoids
- Wounds

Effective Applications

Goldenrod's Latin name, *Solidago*, means "to make whole"—such an appropriate name for this plant! Goldenrod has notable anti-inflammatory and antiseptic actions that make it excellent for wound healing, both on the skin and in the digestive tract. Goldenrod is especially helpful for oral abscesses and wounds, heartburn, and stomach ulcers.

Like many other astringents, goldenrod has a tonifying influence on the mucous membranes. This helps dry up drippy, runny noses, weepy eyes, and phlegmy lungs and, combined with goldenrod's antihistamine action, is part of the reason goldenrod is so helpful for seasonal allergies.

Goldenrod has a particular affinity for aiding in kidney and urinary tract health; one reason is that the volatile oils in goldenrod are eliminated via the urinary system in their whole form—their antimicrobial action is still working even as the goldenrod is leaving your body! For those with chronic UTIs, a daily regimen of goldenrod tea can be a powerful form of defense.

Katja and her daughter, Amber, have had braces for the past year, and both have found goldenrod very soothing to the tissue irritation that is a part of that experience. Steadily sipping warm goldenrod tea throughout the day is

The astringent and diuretic actions can also help with kidney stones and prostatitis, and the anti-inflammatory action is very soothing to affected tissues.

Topical applications of goldenrod (infused into oil) are quite relaxant to the muscles and particularly soothing to lower-back pain.

Recommended Dosage

Goldenrod makes an absolutely delicious tea, and because so much of its action is rooted in kidney support, tea is a great way to work with this plant. Goldenrod can be taken as needed to soothe irritations, but for chronic and long-standing ailments, it's best to have 3 to 4 cups of goldenrod tea daily.

Important Considerations

Though often blamed for seasonal allergy flare-ups, goldenrod is actually insect-pollinated: Its pollen is too heavy to be carried in the air. It is in fact the pollen from ragweed, which flowers at the same time, that is responsible for allergy symptoms—and goldenrod can actually function as an antidote!

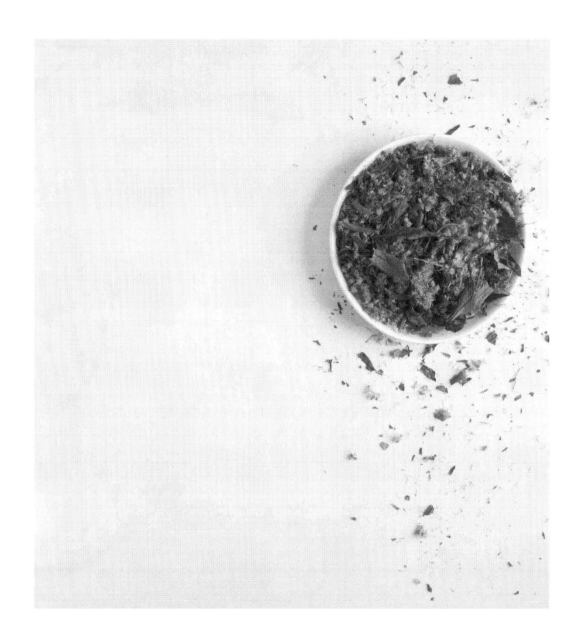

Kelp_ Alaria esculenta

Qualities: cooling, moistening, relaxant

Taste: salty, sweet

Family: Alariaceae

Medicinal parts: lamina (leaves)

Actions: cardiac tonic, demulcent, emollient, mineral-rich nutritive, musculoskeletal tonic, thyroid restorative, vulnerary

Common Preparations

By far the best way to prepare kelp is in a long-simmered broth. Kelp can also be prepared in tea, as a vinegar extract, and in food.

Ideal for Addressing

* ADD/ADHD
* Anxiety
* Arthritis
* Breast fibroids and cysts
* Heartburn/reflux/GERD
* Heart palpitations
* Hypothyroidism
* Menopause/andropause
* Pain management
* Plantar fasciitis
* Rash
* Sprains and strains

Effective Applications

One of kelp's strongest attributes is its high nutritional content. This is increasingly more important as the quality of our soils degrades— and, with it, levels of vitamins and minerals in our land vegetables. This super-food aspect of kelp plays a critical role in every facet of its application.

Kelp can be helpful for nervous issues such as ADD and anxiety because of its high mineral and nutrient content and its soothing, moistening action. Kelp is also beneficial to the adrenal glands (and the entire endocrine system), which can be a significant factor in both ADD and anxiety. It may seem overly simple just to "nourish" these ailments away, but it's actually a surprisingly effective part of a protocol for these and other nervous system issues.

This nutritive action, and in particular the thyroid-boosting effect of kelp, is very helpful for reproductive issues, especially around menstruation, menopause, and andropause. These issues are all about endocrine function, and kelp's high iodine content, among other things, can keep the whole system running more smoothly.

Kelp can be applied topically to wounds for an anti-infective, wound-healing action.

It's also fantastic for sprains and strains, both to speed the healing through anti-inflammatory action and to reduce pain. This is appropriate for both external wounds and skin irritations and irritation in the digestive tract.

A few years ago, Katja broke her toe while leading an herb walk barefoot. As soon as we returned home, we rehydrated some dried kelp and wrapped it around the toe and foot. This not only sped up the healing of the break considerably, but also wiped out the pain. As long as the seaweed was on her foot, nothing hurt!

Recommended Dosage

Kelp is a vegetable, so even more than most herbs, we think about it in terms of serving sizes. Kelp is a very complex plant, and many of its constituents take time to break down, which is why broth is such a good way to take it. If it's a new flavor for you, there's another benefit: Although there will be a "seaweedy" or "fishy" smell for the first 10 to 15 minutes, this dissipates quickly and the resulting broth does not retain the smell or flavor. It's also easy to add a handful of confetti-size pieces to a pot of rice—the result is very mild and easy for seaweed "beginners."

Important Considerations

Buy kelp in its whole, unprocessed, simply dried form, and cook it yourself for the most nutrition and medicinal benefit. It's important to consider the origin of your seaweed, as so much of our oceans is now polluted. Check the Resources section for reputable sources.

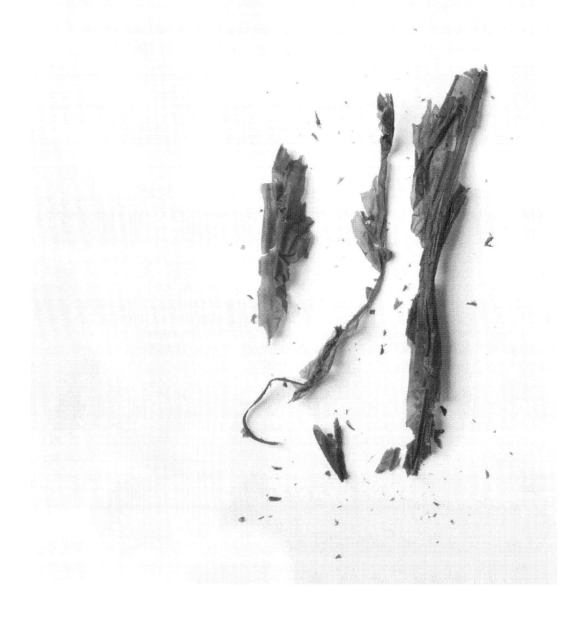

Licorice Glycyrrhiza glabra

Qualities: warming, moistening, relaxant

Taste: sweet

Family: Fabaceae

Medicinal parts: rhizome (root)

Actions: adaptogen, antitussive, demulcent, emollient, expectorant, hepatoprotective, sialagogue, stomach tonic

Common Preparations

Licorice can be prepared as either an infusion or a decoction, for tea or topical application. It can also be tinctured, infused into oil, and made into a salve.

Ideal for Addressing

* Arthritis
* Asthma
* Fatigue
* Food sensitivities
* Hangover
* Heartburn/reflux/GERD
* IBS/IBD/ulcerative colitis
* Inflammation
* Leaky gut
* Sore throat
* Stomach ulcer/gastritis

Effective Applications

Licorice has a moistening effect, which makes it an excellent remedy for dry, itchy, irritated conditions throughout the body. This includes everything from eczema to heartburn and even the "dry," frazzled feeling of being exhausted and stressed.

Add licorice's strong anti-inflammatory action, and you have a plant perfectly suited to treat conditions like stomach ulcers, IBS, and ulcerative colitis, with painful irritation in the digestive tract. Licorice not only reduces inflammation but also helps heal the mucous membranes in the digestive tract, making it an important part of Gut-Heal Tea. Licorice can also simply be paired with self-heal or goldenrod for this effect, as well.

Licorice helps moisten dry lungs and sore throats, and its antitussive action helps relieve dry, unproductive coughs. Combined with ginger, this can be a perfect formula for alleviating winter discomfort. For those who live in dry climates and feel frequently dehydrated, a formula of licorice and linden or marshmallow can provide great relief.

Licorice has strong liver-protective effects, restoring damaged liver tissue and reducing inflammatory irritations. Licorice also strongly supports the adrenal glands and the endocrine system and is excellent for addressing chronic or long-standing conditions, including adrenal exhaustion and endocrine imbalance.

When applied topically, licorice has a strong anti-inflammatory effect. This allows your body's response to itchy, irritated issues such as bites, stings, rashes, eczema, and psoriasis to work more effectively, so you may not need to apply synthetic cortisone topically. An important plant for the skin, licorice moistens skin while calming itching and inflammation.

Recommended Dosage

Licorice has a very strong, sweet flavor and is best suited to multi-herb formulations. It can also be an excellent addition to a formula that leans too far to the dry side. In formula, licorice can be taken 3 to 4 times a day, either as tea or tincture. Licorice is more soluble in water than alcohol, so it is best in tinctures with lower alcohol content or as a strong decoction preserved with 20 percent alcohol. Licorice can be applied topically multiple times daily, as needed.

Important Considerations

Licorice is not recommended in high doses for those with high blood pressure. Deglycyrrhizinated licorice (DGL) products sidestep this concern.

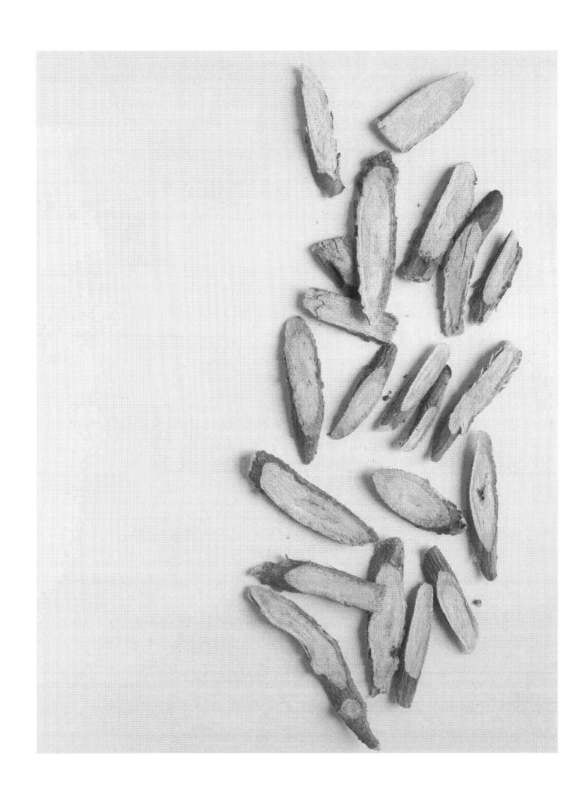

<u>Linden</u> Tilia spp.

Qualities: cooling, moistening, relaxant
Taste: sweet, mildly salty, mildly aromatic
Family: Malvaceae
Medicinal parts: leaves and flowers
Actions: anodyne, anti-inflammatory, anxiolytic, aromatic, demulcent, hypotensive, nervine, relaxant, diaphoretic, sedative, sialagogue

Common Preparations

Linden can be prepared in either a hot or cold infusion, for tea or topical application. Linden can also be made into a tincture, elixir, or infused into wine or mead.

Ideal for Addressing

- ADD/ADHD
- Anxiety
- Burns and sunburn
- Depression
- Heartburn/reflux/GERD
- Heart palpitations
- High blood pressure/hypertension
- Insomnia
- PMS
- Stress

Effective Applications

Linden is helpful for high blood pressure, heart palpitations, arrhythmia, angina, tightness and dryness in the chest, and those with histories of heart attack, stroke, and cardiovascular surgery. Part of this soothing, restorative effect comes from its ability to relax the nervous system, reducing stress on the heart, and part of it comes from direct restorative action on the heart and cardiovascular system in general.

For the emotional heart and nervous system, linden has broad application. Its gentle yet effective cooling nervine action is perfect for anxiety, nervous tension, insomnia, and agitation. Linden is particularly suited to mitigate the side effects of drying, stimulating medications like Adderall and Ritalin and is well tolerated in children and adults alike.

Linden is soothing to nerve pain wherever it appears in the body. Intestinal pain from indigestion and allergies to foods, systemic nerve pain from fibromyalgia and multiple sclerosis, tension headaches, tense menstrual cramps, nerve damage due to injury, and nerve pains due to viruses, including herpes, are all calmed by linden. Imagine being able to rub lotion into "fried and frazzled" nerves—that's exactly how linden can help!

We call linden "a hug in a mug." When what you really need more than anything is a hug and someone to tell you that everything is going to work out all right, linden can give it to you! Sure, it's just a cup of tea, but linden's relaxing and soothing powers can really change your whole outlook on life—and sometimes that's exactly what we need.

Recommended Dosage

A cup of linden tea is soothing in the moment, but for chronic or long-standing issues, plan to make linden a supportive part of your daily life. Three to 4 cups a day, in formula or by itself, is a soothing form of self-care. For a more moistening effect, prepare linden as a cold infusion, or steep it covered overnight: The water starts out hot but cools overnight, so you get the benefit of both the hot water–soluble and cold water–soluble constituents.

Important Considerations

Linden leaves and flowers are very safe for all people.

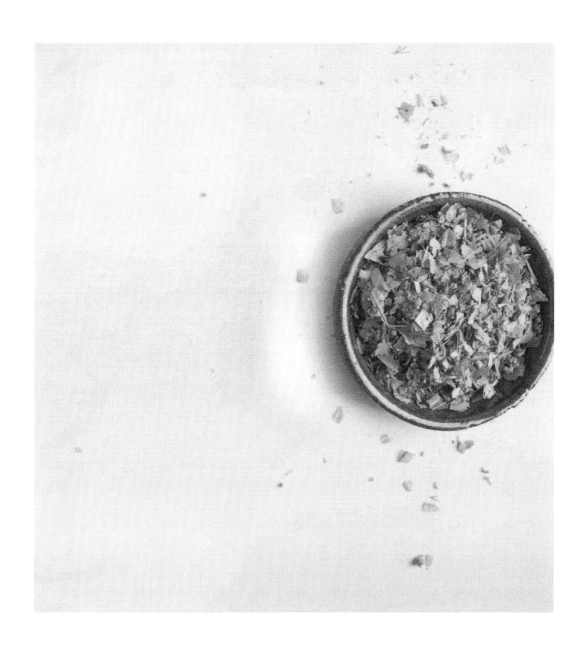

Marshmallow Althaea officinalis

Qualities: cooling, moistening, relaxant

Taste: sweet, salty, bland

Family: Malvaceae

Medicinal parts: root and leaves

Actions: anti-inflammatory, antimicrobial, demulcent, diuretic, emollient, expectorant, nutritive, sialagogue, vulnerary

Common Preparations

Marshmallow root is most effectively prepared as a cold infusion, which may be drunk or used as a bath, poultice, or compress. The leaf can be added to hot infusions or overnight infusions.

Ideal for Addressing

* Arthritis
* Asthma
* Burns and sunburn
* Cough
* Dry mouth
* Food sensitivities
* Gout
* Hangover
* Headache (dehydration)
* Heartburn/reflux/GERD
* High blood pressure/hypertension
* IBS/IBD/ulcerative colitis
* Indigestion/dyspepsia
* Leaky gut

- Sore throat
- Stomach ulcer/gastritis
- Urinary tract infection (UTI)
- Wounds

Effective Applications

Marshmallow's moistening action is very important for dry constitutions and for people who do not hold on to water well. Perhaps you drink a lot of water but feel like it "goes right through you." Marshmallow helps the water "stick," due to its mucilage and mineral content.

Marshmallow also has pronounced, but often overlooked, antimicrobial, anti-inflammatory, and vulnerary actions, which make it ideal for treating irritations—even ulcers—anywhere in the digestive tract. This action is also soothing and effective in the urinary tract, where marshmallow plays an important role in resolving UTIs and cystitis. Marshmallow's moistening action is also excellent to relieve sore throats and tight, dry coughs and respiratory spasms.

Marshmallow's moistening action is effective topically, too: A soak or spray of cold-infused marshmallow is soothing to dry, red skin, particularly when the irritation is caused by heat, salt, or sun damage. Topical applications of marshmallow are also appropriate for treating burns and wounds, soothing inflammation, combating infection, and stimulating the healing processes. Historically, marshmallow was used for problems as severe as sepsis and gangrene!

Recommended Dosage

Marshmallow can be applied topically or taken internally as needed for acute irritation until the problem resolves. For longer-term issues and chronic dehydration, make marshmallow a part of your daily routine. Drink a cup or pint of the thicker cold infusion to soothe painful internal issues such as heartburn and stomach ulcers, or add a half cup of cold infusion to your water bottle each time you refill it to combat dehydration.

Important Considerations

Because of the coating action in the digestive tract, very thick, mucilaginous infusions of marshmallow root can inhibit absorption of medications taken at the same time; take medications separately from marshmallow by at least two hours.

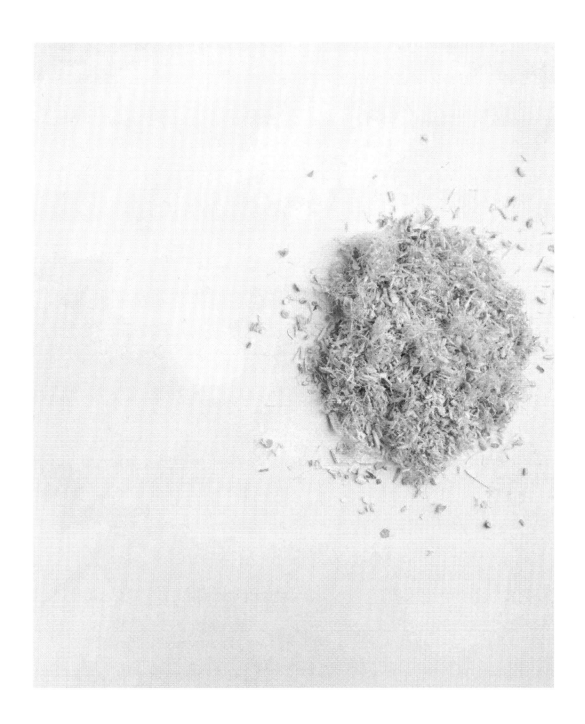

Meadowsweet Filipendula ulmaria

Qualities: cooling, drying, tonifying
Taste: astringent, sweet
Family: Rosaceae
Medicinal parts: leaves and flowers
Actions: anodyne, anti-inflammatory, antimicrobial, aromatic, astringent, diuretic, nervine, vulnerary

Common Preparations

Meadowsweet can be infused for tea or topical applications. Meadowsweet can also be prepared as a tincture or elixir.

Ideal for Addressing

* Abscess
* Back pain
* Diarrhea
* Food sensitivities
* Headache
* Heartburn/reflux/GERD
* IBS/IBD/ulcerative colitis
* Indigestion/dyspepsia
* Joint pain
* Leaky gut
* Pain management
* Receding gums
* Stomach ulcer/gastritis
* Rash (weeping)

Effective Applications

Meadowsweet is a delicious, soothing herb for addressing hot, inflamed conditions, whether that's an irritated, weepy rash, a wound or abscess in the mouth, or irritation and inflammation in the digestive tract or throughout the body. Meadowsweet not only speeds healing and recovery time but also helps relieve pain, due to its salicylate content. Unlike aspirin—acetylsalicylic acid, which can cause ulcers—meadowsweet does not damage the digestive tract, because the salicylates are not converted to their free acid form until they reach the liver. And, in fact, meadowsweet is tremendously effective for resolving ulcers: Not only can it relieve the pain, but the anti-inflammatory and astringent actions help the ulcer heal much faster, too.

The astringent action of meadowsweet is also very effective for diarrhea, as well as edema and cystitis.

Cooling and anti-inflammatory, meadowsweet is especially well suited for treating rheumatoid arthritis symptoms and headaches that feel hot and pounding.

Meadowsweet is another herb that has been very helpful for Katja and her daughter, Amber, in their experience with orthodontics. Meadowsweet is very soothing to the irritation caused by the braces, and helps promote speedy healing, as well. When there was a lot of discomfort, Katja would often just hold a mouthful of warm meadowsweet tea for several minutes, swallow, and immediately do it again.

Recommended Dosage

Meadowsweet tea can be taken as needed, until the problem resolves. It's a delicious tea, and it formulates well with other herbs, so include it in any formula when you're looking for that cooling, anti-inflammatory action.

Important Considerations

Avoid meadowsweet if you are allergic to aspirin.

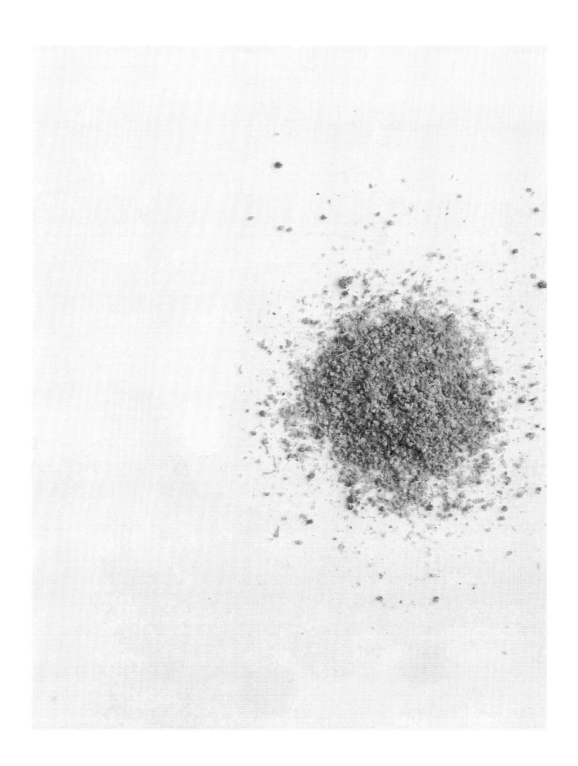

Milk Thistle *Silybum marianum*

Qualities: cooling, moistening, relaxant

Taste: nutty, salty, sweet

Family: Asteraceae

Medicinal parts: seeds

Actions: alterative, anti-inflammatory, emollient, expectorant, hepatic, hepatoprotective

Common Preparations

Milk thistle is most commonly taken in capsule form. It can also be powdered and added to food or smoothies.

Ideal for Addressing

* Acne
* Allergies
* Constipation
* Detox
* Eczema/dermatitis
* Endometriosis
* Hangover
* Hypothyroidism
* Menopause/andropause
* PCOS
* Rash

Effective Applications

An important remedy for the liver, milk thistle has a unique threefold action. It provides nourishment specifically for liver tissue, protects liver cells from damage, and stimulates the regeneration of already damaged liver cells. Milk thistle is also very gentle on the body. Because of its gentleness and strong anti-inflammatory action, milk thistle is an ideal remedy for all kinds of liver problems, including states of acute and chronic inflammation.

Milk thistle is an important herb for people who are chronically stressed, sleep deprived, and overworked, whose high levels of adrenaline and cortisol put an added load on the liver. Milk thistle is also excellent support for insulin-resistant and hormonally imbalanced bodies, as these states also add to the liver's already large workload. This applies to people taking pharmaceuticals, alcohol, and other drugs as well: Anytime the liver has extra detoxification work to do, think milk thistle! Many times, this extra load on the liver shows up on the skin in the form of acne, rashes, or eczema—consider milk thistle in these situations.

Milk thistle is particularly handy for kids in puberty, which is a time of heavy load on the liver. Puberty means lots of hormones for the liver to break down, and that can lead to acne. Plus, many teenagers eat diets higher in sugar, or turn to caffeine to manage late nights of homework—two things the liver has to clear out of the system. Milk thistle is a quick fix for teens because it can be taken in capsules—no extra work required! The same goes for menopause and andropause, which present many of the same issues, just a few decades later.

Milk thistle is a fantastic hangover recovery herb—whether it's a hangover from alcohol, sugar, or too much caffeine. If you are heading to a party, take two milk thistle capsules before you go and two more when you get home. Remember to stay hydrated! The next morning, take two more: Hangover symptoms will be drastically reduced or may not happen at all!

Recommended Dosage

Although we usually much prefer to work with herbs in tea or other liquid preparations, milk thistle is an herb that is very effective as a capsule. This can be handy, especially because supporting the liver is important for almost every ailment. You can have a quart of tea daily that is specifically targeted to the recovery you're trying to make, and just add milk thistle capsules for extra liver support. We typically recommend two capsules daily for background support and two twice daily for liver-specific issues.

Important Considerations

A very safe herb, milk thistle is effective in capsule form and has no known drug interactions. Heavy use may have a mild laxative effect.

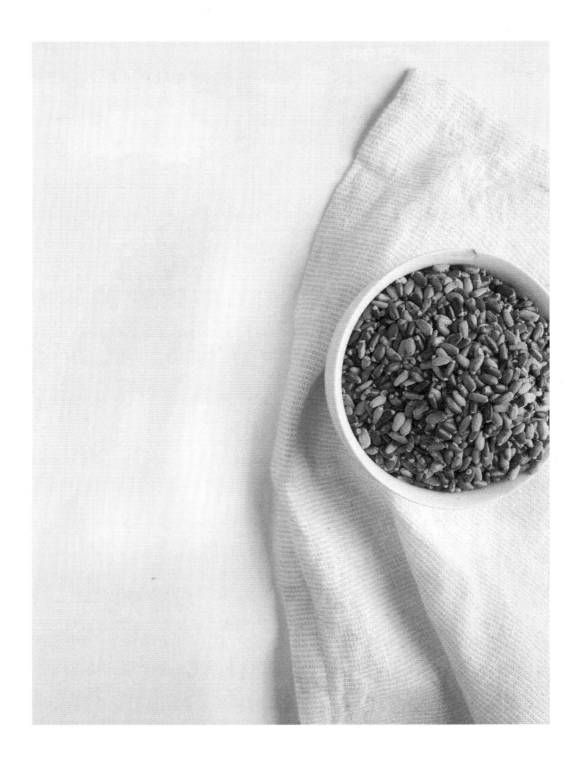

<u>Mullein</u> Verbascum thapsus, V. densiflorum

Qualities: cooling, drying, tonifying

Taste: salty, mucilaginous

Family: Scrophulariaceae

Medicinal parts: leaves, flowers, root

Actions: anodyne, anticatarrhal, anti-inflammatory, antimicrobial, moistening expectorant, nervous sedative, respiratory relaxant, urinary and connective tissue tonic

Common Preparations

Mullein leaves can be prepared as tea or tincture, and applied topically. Mullein root can be made into a decoction or tincture. Mullein flowers are typically infused into oil and can also be infused for tea. Any of the plant parts can be infused into oil to make a salve. Mullein leaves can also be smoked.

Ideal for Addressing

- Allergies
- Asthma
- Back pain
- Cough
- Ear infection/earache
- Incontinence

Effective Applications

A moistening expectorant and respiratory relaxant, mullein leaf is particularly indicated for dry, hacking coughs. Mullein leaf loosens and moistens mucus in the lungs, making it easier to expel, and is particularly helpful for unproductive coughs.

Mullein is very effective for loosening and bringing up the thick, "baked on" mucus that results from smoking cigarettes and is helpful for keeping smokers' lungs clear. Mullein can also be smoked and can be slowly substituted for tobacco over a period of time while trying to quit smoking cigarettes.

Additionally, mullein helps expectorate any environmental contaminants inhaled into the lungs, which cause congestive problems and infections: Construction workers, painters, miners, firemen, mechanics, potters—anyone who works in a dry, dusty, or chemical-laden environment would benefit from a quart of mullein tea daily.

Mullein leaf also has anti-inflammatory action, with particular affinity to the joints and skeleton, and is restorative to connective tissues, including the spinal discs. Mullein can be applied topically to injuries or areas with chronic pain.

Mullein root is relaxing to the nervous system, yet exerts a tonifying effect on the bladder. Incontinence and frequent urination can be reduced with a tincture of mullein root.

Mullein flower–infused olive oil dropped into the ears soothes the pain of earache, helps clear the infection, and loosens stuck or compacted earwax. Be sure to warm it slightly for comfort.

Recommended Dosage

Mullein leaf makes a tasty tea and can be taken daily, alone or in formula, for lung support and more. Mullein root is not typically sold commercially, but you do not need to wildcraft large quantities, as root tincture is very effective at lower doses—1 dropperful 2 to 3 times daily is sufficient. Three to four root balls should be sufficient to make enough tincture for a year. Mullein flower oil can be made in small quantities, as you will only use 1 to 2 drops per ear as needed.

Important Considerations

Mullein leaves are covered in tiny hairs, which can be irritating: Strain the tea well.

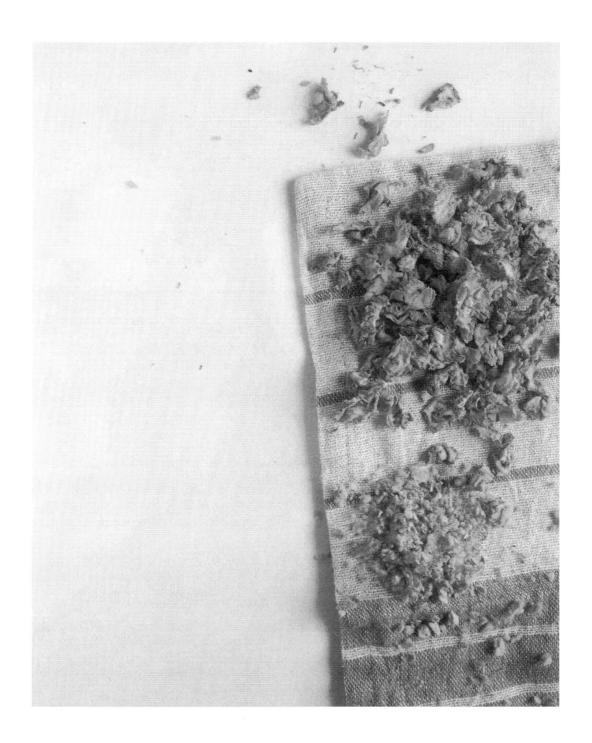

Nettle Urtica dioica

Qualities: cooling, drying, tonifying
Taste: earthy, salty, umami
Family: Urticaceae
Medicinal parts: leaves, root
Actions: alterative, diuretic, kidney tonic, nutritive

Common Preparations

Nettle leaves can be long infused for a high-mineral tea, or added to soup and stew. Nettle roots are most commonly tinctured or taken as a capsule.

Ideal for Addressing

- Allergies
- BPH/prostatitis
- Detox
- Endometriosis
- Gout
- Incontinence
- Kidney stones
- Menopause/andropause
- PCOS
- Rash
- Urinary tract infection (UTI)

Effective Applications

Nettle tea is, above all, a multivitamin and mineral supplement in a teacup! One of the most mineral-rich land plants, nettle, when taken regularly, can resolve many issues resulting from the lack of minerals in modern diets. Often, it's not that nettle is an herbal medicine required for a specific ailment but that the ailment was due to "nettle deficiency"—a lack of vitamin- and mineral-rich foods in the diet.

Nettle leaf is not just nourishing, it also has specific beneficial effect on the kidneys, and through them the endocrine system. This makes nettle essential support for issues that affect the urinary system, like gout, UTI, and kidney stones, and also for hormonally based issues, such as endometriosis and PCOS. Nettle leaf can be very supportive through the phases of menopause, as well.

Nettle has a fairly strong astringent action, especially in the pelvic region, which makes it a perfect support for BPH and prostatitis, as well as incontinence. However, for people who run dry, the astringent action can be aggravating over time: Formulate it with linden or marshmallow to balance the dryness.

Nettle is one of the best supports for seasonal allergies—not only because of its strong kidney-supporting actions, but also because nettle can stimulate the liver's antihistamine production, and it even has its own antihistamine constituents to contribute to the cause! A quart of long-infused nettle tea daily, starting 1 to 2 weeks before your usual allergy season, is a great way to get this support, but freeze-dried nettle capsules will also do the trick.

Believe it or not, the sting from fresh nettles can also be medicine! The tiny hairs are loaded with formic acid, which causes topical irritation—but also causes the body to flush the area, which makes that sting very effective for relieving arthritis symptoms.

Recommended Dosage

Nettle leaves are food; think of them in serving-size quantities. A quart of long-infused tea daily is an excellent way to get the full benefit of nettle leaves. This can be helpful when you just don't have time to incorporate fresh vegetables into your diet, or you just need the extra support nettle can provide. Nettle root can be taken in tincture or capsules daily for support of long-term genitourinary issues. If the effect is too drying over time, 1 to 2 cups of linden or marshmallow infusion daily can provide balancing moisture.

Important Considerations

Fresh nettle leaf can raise a temporary rash on the skin. This typically passes quickly, and the effect is neutralized by drying or cooking the nettle.

If you take thyroid medication, wait 2 hours after taking it before consuming long infusions of nettle. *Do not take nettle leaf in high doses if you take pharmaceutical blood thinners*.

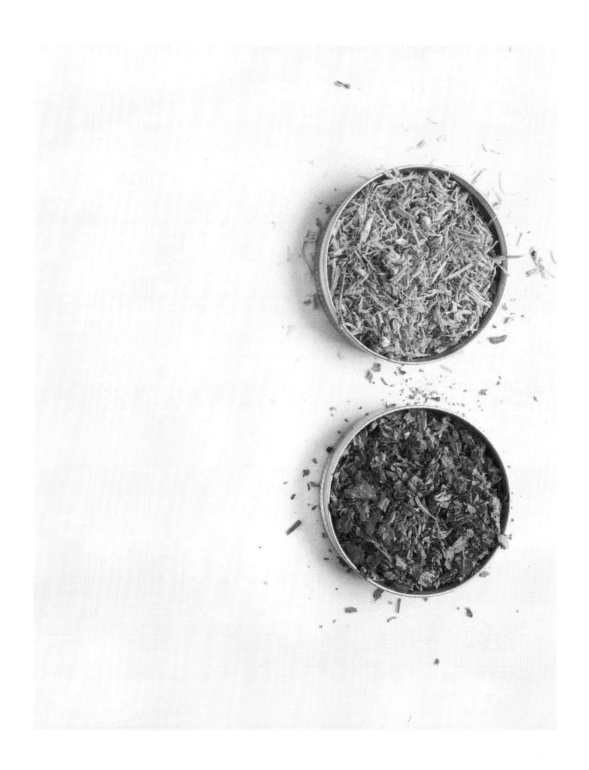

<u>Peppermint</u> Mentha × piperita

Qualities: warming, drying, relaxant

Taste: aromatic, pungent, minty

Family: Lamiaceae

Medicinal parts: leaves and flowers

Actions: anticatarrhal, antiemetic, anti-inflammatory, antimicrobial, antispasmodic, aromatic, carminative, cholagogue, stimulating diaphoretic

Common Preparations

Peppermint leaves can be infused into water for tea or into oil for salves. Peppermint can also be prepared as a steam.

Ideal for Addressing

* Arthritis
* Bites and stings
* Bloating
* Burns and sunburn
* Fever
* Food sensitivities
* IBS/IBD/ulcerative colitis
* Indigestion/dyspepsia
* Leaky gut
* Muscle soreness/post-workout recovery
* Nausea

Effective Applications

Peppermint has a relaxing action throughout the body, which can be helpful in the digestive system to relieve gas and bloating, and colic in children. This relaxing action can also be effective for muscle soreness, especially when applied topically. In fact, peppermint can even relax the mind in stressful situations—but it doesn't dull the senses: Peppermint stimulates the flow of oxygen to the brain, so while the end effect is relaxing, the mind is sharpened.

Peppermint's volatile oils, much like thyme and sage, are antimicrobial and very effective in a steam against respiratory infections. The relaxing action of peppermint also helps release fever, and because the flavor often appeals to children, this is a very handy plant for sick little ones.

Like nettle and dandelion, peppermint is high in minerals. And the widely appealing flavor makes peppermint a welcome addition to the somewhat grassy flavor of the other high-mineral herbs. Add rosehips for a complete multivitamin in a teapot!

There can be debate about whether peppermint is warming or cooling—after all, it leaves a refreshing, cooling feeling in the mouth. Peppermint is actually warming: It stimulates blood flow and metabolic activity where applied. But it also stimulates cold-sensing nerves, which yields the impression of cold. And because it relaxes muscles and blood vessels, it allows heat to escape the body, cooling a fever.

Recommended Dosage

Peppermint can be taken freely as tea as desired. Its pleasant flavor makes an excellent cover for less palatable herbs.

Important Considerations

Large amounts of peppermint may relax the lower esophageal sphincter and induce heartburn in susceptible individuals.

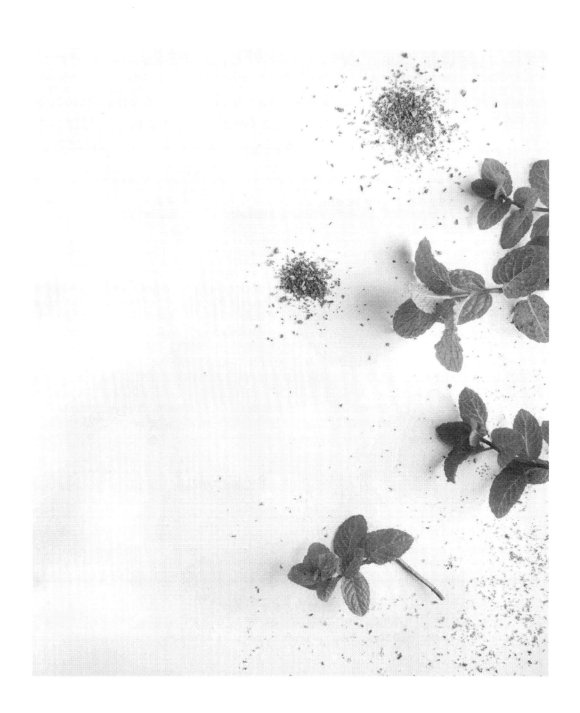

Pine Pinus strobus

Qualities: warming, drying, tonifying
Taste: aromatic
Family: Pinaceae
Medicinal parts: leaves
Actions: anticatarrhal, antimicrobial, antiseptic, aromatic, astringent, diuretic, expectorant, vulnerary

Common Preparations

White pine can be prepared as tea, tincture, or elixir. Pine resin can be made into a salve.

Ideal for Addressing

- Abscess
- Bronchitis/chest cold/pneumonia
- Cold and flu
- Cough
- Depression
- Gingivitis
- Immune support
- Receding gums
- Sinusitis/stuffy nose
- Wounds

Effective Applications

Pine is most commonly associated with immune support and respiratory ailments. The aromatic, volatile oils in all conifer trees are directly antiseptic to the respiratory system, helping kill invading pathogens. As tea, pine warms the respiratory system and acts as an expectorant to move phlegm up and out of the lungs. Pine makes an effective and enjoyable steam for respiratory infections and is a great choice if a thyme steam feels too intensely warming (see Thyme).

Pine is also a mood-boosting, uplifting remedy. Long walks in the woods have been shown scientifically to reduce stress, aid in depression, and have many other health benefits, which has led to the recent fascination with "forest bathing." But our modern lifestyles don't always offer the time we need to get those benefits. Fortunately, because some of those actions come from the volatile oils of pine trees, a steamy, hot cup of pine needle tea can bring many of the same benefits right to you, wherever you are.

Pine resin is an excellent remedy for wound healing. Strongly antiseptic, pine resin prevents infection, and its vulnerary actions stimulate healing. Pine Resin Salve is indispensable in a first aid kit, though on the trail, the resin can even be applied in its natural (sticky!) state.

After gathering pine resin, it can be very difficult to wash it off your hands. Use oil instead of water—the resin is oil soluble, and comes right off when you "wash" your hands with oil.

Recommended Dosage

Pine needle tea can be taken freely as needed, or as desired for its deliciousness! Pine resin salve can be applied to shallow wounds multiple times daily until the wound heals.

Important Considerations

There are many species of pine trees, and many have herbal applications, but some do not. To be sure you have white pine, check the "bundles" of pine needles—if long, flexible needles grow in bundles of five, you have white pine!

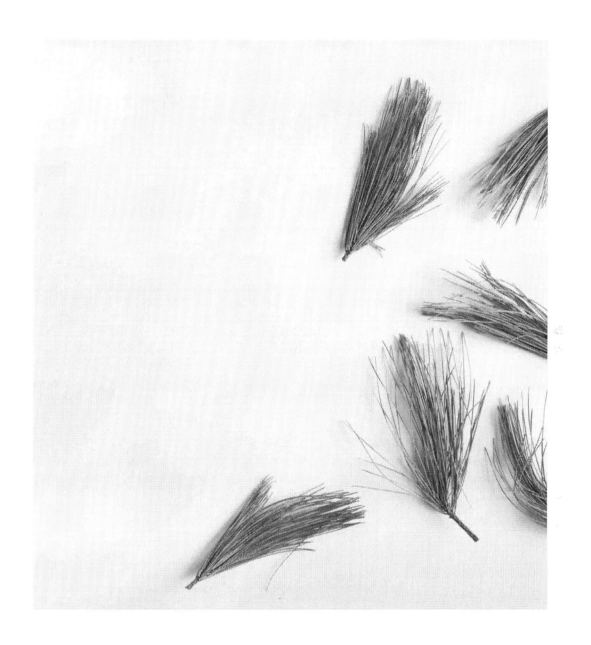

<u>Plantain</u> Plantago major, rugelii, lanceolata

Qualities: cooling, moistening, tonifying
Taste: slightly bitter, earthy
Family: Plantaginaceae
Medicinal parts: leaves
Actions: anti-inflammatory, antimicrobial, astringent, demulcent, emollient, expectorant, hepatoprotective, vulnerary

Common Preparations

Plantain leaves can be prepared as a tea or tincture for internal and topical use. The leaves can also be infused into oil for lotion or salve.

Ideal for Addressing

- Abscess and gingivitis
- Allergies
- Athlete's foot/fungal skin infections
- Bites and stings
- Burns and sunburn
- Diarrhea
- Eczema and dermatitis
- Food sensitivities
- Hangover
- Herpes/cold sores/chickenpox
- IBS/IBD/ulcerative colitis
- Indigestion/dyspepsia
- Leaky gut
- Rash

- Receding gums
- Stomach ulcer/gastritis
- Wounds
- Yeast infection

Effective Applications

Plantain is a vulnerary, promoting the growth of new cells to speed wound healing. This action applies both to the skin and the entire digestive tract lining, making plantain a very handy plant to have around. Everything from eczema to wounds and abrasions to ulcers and leaky gut heal faster with plantain.

Plantain is another of our very strong biofilm-disrupting herbs, which means it can help break up infection even in antibiotic-resistant situations. Combining plantain with other antimicrobial herbs, or even with pharmaceutical antibiotics, makes a much more effective remedy than either one alone.

Plantain also has a gentle astringent action, which, combined with the ability to break up biofilms, makes it excellent in situations such as gingivitis or dental abscesses: It is able to break up and drain the infection and tighten the gums.

Plantain is also liver protective. This is handy in mundane situations such as a hangover, but it also enhances plantain's antimicrobial capability, as the liver plays such an important role in fighting infection.

Recommended Dosage

Plantain can be applied topically several times daily for wounds or other topical irritations until the situation clears. As tea, especially for digestive issues, 3 to 4 cups daily, alone or in formula (see Gut-Heal Tea), is appropriate.

Important Considerations

The herb plantain has no relationship to the small banana-like fruit, except the same name.

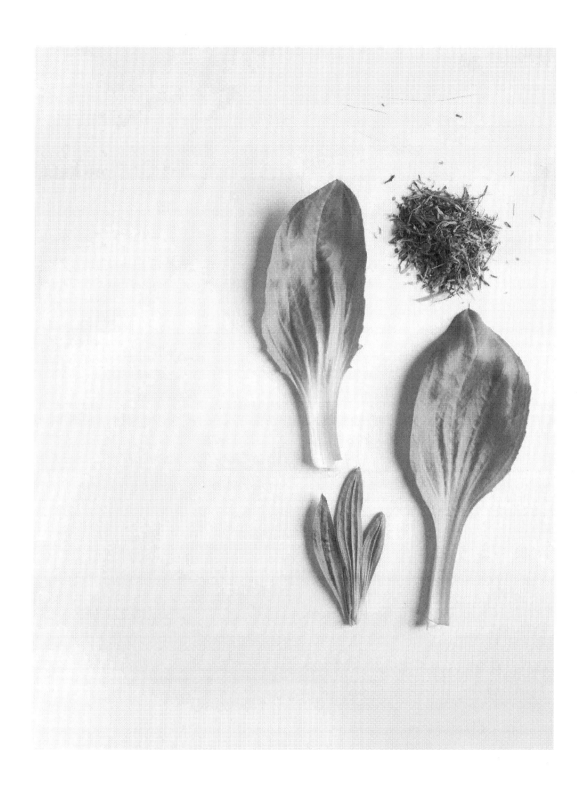

Rose Rosa canina, multiflora, rugosa

Qualities: cooling, drying, tonifying

Taste: sweet, aromatic, astringent, sour

Family: Rosaceae

Medicinal parts: flowers, hips (fruits), root

Actions: petals—antimicrobial, aromatic, astringent, exhilarant, nervine, refrigerant, vulnerary; hips—nutritive, refrigerant; root—astringent, refrigerant

Common Preparations

Rose can be infused into water for tea or a topical application, or tinctured in vinegar or alcohol. Rose can also be infused into oil for salve. Rosehips can be made as tea or prepared as food. Rose water can be applied directly to the skin and taken internally. Rose petals can be infused into honey to enjoy on its own or for blending elixirs. Rose roots are most commonly prepared as tincture.

Ideal for Addressing

* Acne
* Anxiety
* Bites and stings
* Burns and sunburn
* Cholesterol management
* Depression
* Diarrhea
* Eczema and dermatitis
* Edema
* Heart palpitations

- High blood pressure/hypertension
- Insomnia
- Rash
- Stress
- Varicose veins and hemorrhoids

Effective Applications

Rose petals are astringent and promote the growth of new cells, and rose roots are more strongly astringent than the petals or leaves, which means rose is particularly effective at drying and healing wet or weeping wounds when applied topically. In fact, rose is excellent for a whole range of skin issues, from eczema to acne to keeping skin looking healthy and vibrant. Rose water—the same that is often used in cooking—or rose petals infused into water, makes an excellent wound wash, soak for rashes, and face wash.

That astringent and healing action is also appropriate in the digestive tract for diarrhea, leaky gut conditions, gut inflammation, and ulcerations.

Rose makes an excellent topical treatment for any type of burn. The cooling action of rose relieves the painful, hot sensation on contact and helps promote new cell growth. That cooling, anti-inflammatory action works throughout the body as well and is even helpful in stressful and anxiety-inducing situations.

In the wild, rose brambles grow like umbrellas close to the ground, and small, furry creatures scurry among the thorned vines to hide from predator animals. Rose can also provide this protection in times when we humans feel emotionally vulnerable.

Rose has a particularly uplifting effect on the heart, both physiologically and emotionally. The petals provide the relaxing effect, and the hips are high in nourishing antioxidants to help keep the entire cardiovascular system healthy.

Recommended Dosage

Rose hips can be enjoyed regularly as food or as a nutritional tea. Blend with other nutritive herbs such as nettles, dandelion, and even seaweed for a tasty, high-vitamin tea. Rose petals can be added freely to tea, but they have a bitter flavor if steeped for too long, so blend with herbs that have strong flavors, such as tulsi or mint. A spoonful of rosewater can be added to any tea for an uplifting effect or even just to hot water all by itself! For skin care, apply rose water frequently throughout the day until the issue resolves or daily for routine skin care.

Important Considerations

The rose used in herbalism is not the same rose you find at the florist, though those are lovely! For herbalism, the wild varieties are preferable. If you grow roses, it's generally fine to use any of the varieties that have a strong rose scent.

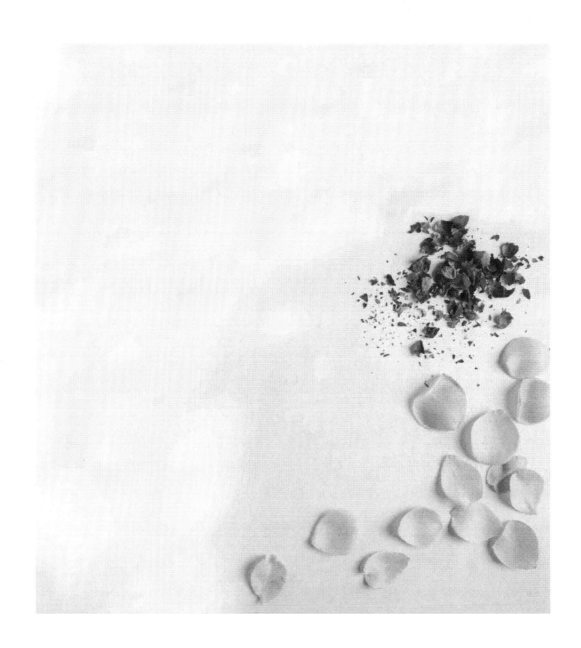

Sage Salvia officinalis

Qualities: warming, drying, tonifying

Taste: aromatic, astringent, bitter, slightly oily

Family: Lamiaceae

Medicinal parts: leaves

Actions: anticatarrhal, antimicrobial, antitussive, aromatic, carminative, circulatory stimulant, diaphoretic, diffusive, hepatic, respiratory nervine

Common Preparations

Sage leaves are often included in cooking, and can be prepared as tea, tincture, or elixir. They can also be added to a steam inhalation or infused into oil for a salve.

Ideal for Addressing

- Abscess and gingivitis
- Acne
- Bronchitis/chest cold/pneumonia
- Cough
- Edema
- Fever
- Menopause/andropause
- Menstrual cycle irregularities
- PMS
- Receding gums
- Sinusitis/stuffy nose
- Sore throat
- Stress

Effective Applications

Warming, somewhat bitter, and astringent, sage stimulates digestive secretions and is particularly effective at breaking down dietary fats —which is why it's so commonly included in recipes for roast meats and sausage. Sage is an important herb for people who have trouble digesting meat and fat.

Sage is antimicrobial in the respiratory tract and is excellent in a steam or as a gargle for sore throats, to fight viruses and loosen mucus, and to reduce coughing. It is particularly effective against the rhinovirus, which causes many colds and sore throats (especially those associated with post-nasal drip).

Long in the past, sage was considered an important herb for nervous system overwhelm, and now, in our modern times, it's coming back into fashion. Sage is particularly effective for people who feel overwhelmed with everything that must be done but don't see any way to get help. Blended with tulsi and betony, sage can make your outlook on an impossible situation much more manageable.

Recommended Dosage

For colds and flu, sage is most effective as a steam or hot tea, employed multiple times a day until the sickness passes. For stress management, 1 to 3 cups of sage tea daily, alone or in combination with other nervous system–supporting herbs, can be very helpful. A tincture or elixir is also a lovely, and speedier, way to work with sage in stressful situations. For improving digestion, sage can be added directly to foods or taken as a tincture before meals. Sage's bitter and liver-stimulating action can be excellent for reproductive system issues, whether taken as tea or tincture.

Important Considerations

Sage is quite drying; for people who run dry, it's best to formulate with moistening herbs such as marshmallow or linden. Sage is not recommended during breastfeeding, unless it is intended to slow or stop milk production.

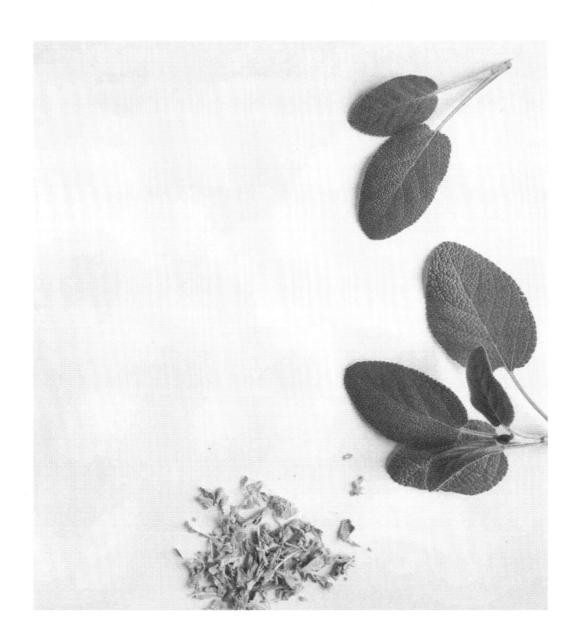

Self-Heal Prunella vulgaris

Qualities: cooling, drying, tonifying
Taste: mildly aromatic, mildly astringent, mildly bitter
Family: Lamiaceae
Medicinal parts: leaves and flowers
Actions: antimicrobial, antiviral, astringent, diuretic, immunomodulator, lymphatic, styptic, vulnerary

Common Preparations

Self-heal leaves and flowers can be infused into water as tea or for topical application, as well as infused into oil for topical use or to make a salve. Tincture and elixir are also effective.

Ideal for Addressing

* Abscess and gingivitis
* Allergies
* Bloating
* BPH/prostatitis
* Breast fibroids and cysts
* Burns and sunburn
* Eczema and dermatitis
* Edema
* Food sensitivities
* Heartburn/reflux/GERD
* Herpes/cold sores/chickenpox
* IBS/IBD/ulcerative colitis
* Inflammation
* Leaky gut

- Stomach ulcer/gastritis
- Wounds

Effective Applications

Self-heal inhibits the binding ability of a virus, so the virus can't replicate. Additionally, self-heal can disrupt biofilms, making bacteria easier to fight. To round it out, self-heal stimulates the lymphatic system—your body's "cleanup crew" during and after an illness. Together, this makes self-heal your first-choice defense for whatever infection you have—even if you don't know what it is! Self-heal doesn't have any known drug interactions, so you can feel free to take it even if you're also on antibiotics.

Self-heal supports kidney health, stimulates lymphatic movement, and has an immune system-modulating effect—which makes it perfect for supporting seasonal allergies. A quart of tea daily, alone or in formula with herbs such as nettle and goldenrod, is a great way to get through allergy season. These actions also are particularly effective against issues with lymphatic stagnation, such as edema, fibroids and cysts, and prostatitis.

Self-heal is excellent for wounds, internally and externally. The antiviral and antibacterial actions help fight infection, the astringency helps stop bleeding, and the vulnerary action helps grow healthy new tissue. Apply topically or drink plenty of tea to combat digestive tract issues, such as stomach ulcers, IBS, and leaky gut.

Self-heal is a delicate, lovely little plant with tremendous medicinal action. We particularly love the way that self-heal reminds us that "gentle" can be potent, and harshness is not required for strong medicine.

Recommended Dosage

Self-heal can be applied topically for skin infections or wound healing, either as a compress or soak, or infused into oil or made into a salve. Apply several times a day until the issue resolves. As tea, self-heal is best taken daily for supporting chronic issues.

Important Considerations

Although self-heal has no known interactions, it is important to *be cautious if you take pharmaceutical blood thinners.*

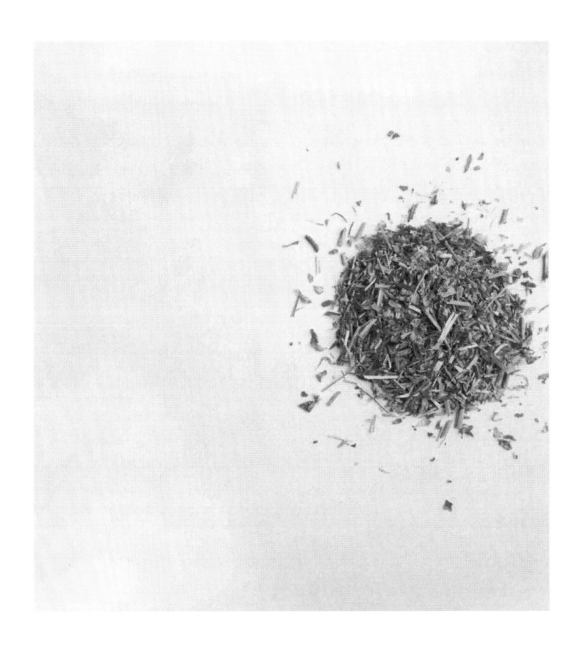

Solomon's Seal Polygonatum biflorum, multiflorum

Qualities: cooling, moistening, relaxant

Taste: sweet, slightly acrid

Family: Asparagaceae

Medicinal parts: rhizome (root)

Actions: anti-inflammatory, antispasmodic, astringent, demulcent, hypotensive, joint lubricant, nutritive, tension modulator, vulnerary

Common Preparations

Solomon's seal roots are best prepared as a tincture for topical and internal use. The roots can also be prepared as an infused oil or a salve or as a decoction.

Ideal for Addressing

- Arthritis
- Back pain
- Incontinence
- Inflammation
- Joint pain
- Plantar fasciitis
- Sprains and strains

Effective Applications

Solomon's seal is moistening and relaxing and can restore lubrication in the joints and rebuild connective tissue, especially where there is inflammation associated with dryness. Solomon's seal can also restore healthy joint function, relaxing overtight connective tissue and moistening overstretched and deteriorating tissue so it returns to its appropriate state. This function is effective whether the condition is chronic, such as arthritis, or acute, such as a sprained ankle, and is especially suited to supporting back injuries.

Solomon's seal taken internally can be helpful for pelvic floor issues such as incontinence. Solomon's seal restores proper levels of tension to the ligaments that hold organs in place, and can support healthy pelvic floor function.

This works emotionally as well: Just as Solomon's seal can help people with joint problems become more flexible and adaptable to changing physical environments, it can also help people become more emotionally and mentally flexible and adaptable. A ▯/▯ dropperful of tincture 2 to 3 times daily can be very helpful for people who want to do this work.

Recommended Dosage

Solomon's seal is a very safe herb, but because it is not abundant in the wild, it is best to work with tincture, because tincture requires less plant matter to make a larger quantity of medicine. Apply topically, alone or in formula, directly to the affected areas as needed, at least 2 to 3 times per day. Solomon's seal can be taken internally to support physiological healing or provide emotional support—▯▯to 1 dropperful is usually sufficient, 3 times daily.

Important Considerations

Some species of Solomon's seal are endangered, and while *Polygonatum biflorum* is not yet endangered, it is considered at risk for overharvesting in the wild. Be especially picky when buying Solomon's seal from a supplier—make sure it was organically cultivated. However, it is an easy herb to grow in a shady spot, and cultivated Solomon's seal is just as effective as wild harvested.

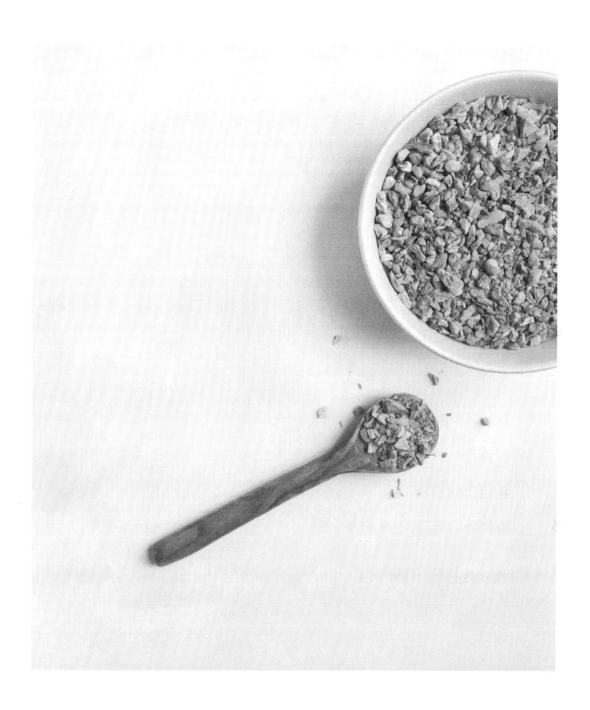

St. John's Wort Hypericum perforatum

Qualities: warming, drying, relaxant
Taste: bitter, aromatic
Family: Hypericaceae
Medicinal parts: leaves and flowers
Actions: alterative, anodyne, anti-inflammatory, antiviral, bitter, exhilarant, hepatic, nerve trophorestorative, nervine, vulnerary

Common Preparations

St. John's wort leaves and flowers can be made into tea, tincture, and elixir. The fresh flowers can be infused into oil for liniments and salves.

Ideal for Addressing

* Acne
* ADD/ADHD
* Depression
* Detox
* Endometriosis
* Hangover
* Herpes/cold sores/chicken pox
* Hypothyroidism
* Inflammation
* Menopause/andropause
* PCOS
* PMS
* Rash
* Seasonal depression

- Sprains and strains
- Stomach ulcer/gastritis
- Stress
- Wounds

Effective Applications

St. John's wort has been touted for depression and can be very effective, especially in situations where there is stagnation and "stuckness." When depression comes along with physical symptoms of constipation or impaired digestion and the feeling of not clearing waste effectively (physically or emotionally), St. John's wort is a great choice. That's because St. John's wort works primarily through the gut and the liver: There is actually much more neurotransmitter activity in the gut than in the brain, so by improving gut function, St. John's wort can affect the emotions we perceive to be in our brains.

One of the liver's most important jobs is daily detox and hormone regulation—it's like the janitorial staff for your body. The word "detox" is often associated with things like environmental toxins and heavy metals, but the far larger part of the daily cycle of detoxification is just the regular clutter of life—much like the dishes, laundry, and vacuuming in your home. Keeping up with the daily clutter improves every aspect of health.

The efficient liver function and gut-brain restoration is also helpful for ADD and ADHD, and kids in puberty—when the neurotransmitters in the gut function efficiently and the liver can keep up with daily detox, it becomes much easier to quiet mental chatter and distraction.

St. John's wort has specific action in restoring nerve function, whether after an injury or viral nerve infection, or repairing chronic inflammation. Combine that with wound healing and soft tissue repair actions, and St. John's wort is the perfect companion for Solomon's seal for topical post-injury support.

St. John's wort is also very effective against "enveloped" viruses, such as those in the herpes family and hepatitis B and C.

Recommended Dosage

Although St. John's wort capsules were popular in the 1990s for addressing depression symptoms, it's the whole herb that can really promote this effect. Tea or tincture, taken regularly, is much more effective than capsules. For topical applications, apply several times daily until the injury completely heals.

Important Considerations

St. John's wort is so effective for improving liver function that it will cause many pharmaceuticals to be cleared from the body too quickly. *Avoid St. John's wort when taking pharmaceuticals that require precise dosing, such as HIV and organ-rejection drugs, or thyroid medication. It should also be avoided with pharmaceuticals that cause withdrawal symptoms upon stopping, such as psychiatric drugs and steroids. If you take pharmaceuticals, check with your pharmacist before trying St. John's wort.*

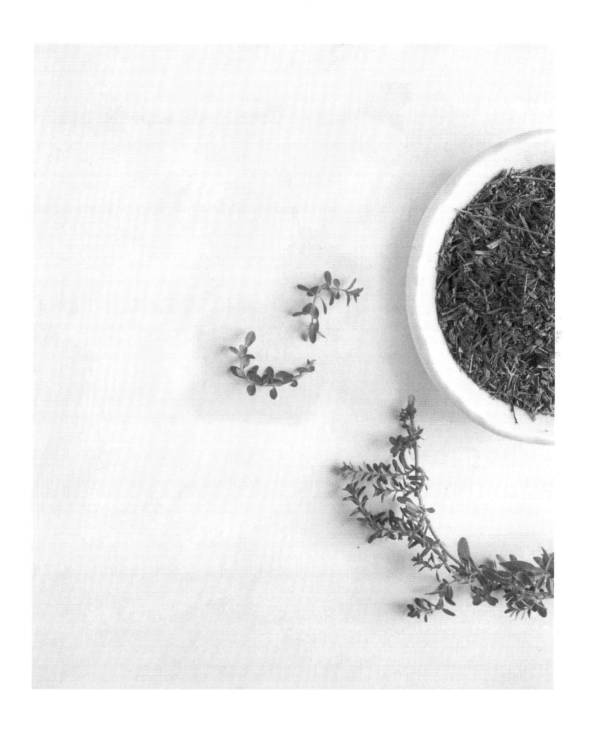

Thyme Thymus vulgaris

Qualities: warming, drying, tonifying
Taste: pungent, aromatic
Family: Lamiaceae
Medicinal parts: leaves and flowers
Actions: anticatarrhal, anti-inflammatory, antimicrobial, antiparasitic, aromatic, carminative, emmenagogue, relaxant, respiratory antimicrobial, stimulating expectorant

Common Preparations

Thyme can be prepared as a steam or infused for tea. Thyme can be infused into apple cider vinegar for topical use or into alcohol as a tincture. It can also be added directly to food.

Ideal for Addressing

* Abscess and gingivitis
* Acne
* Athlete's foot/fungal skin infections
* Bronchitis/chest cold/pneumonia
* Cold and flu
* Cough
* Fever
* Herpes/cold sores/chicken pox
* Immune support
* Sinusitis/stuffy nose
* UTI
* Yeast infection

Effective Applications

Thyme steams are a very important part of our protocol for cold and flu. Thyme's antimicrobial action is in the volatile oils, which are released in hot steam. Breathed deeply into the lungs, thyme steam kills respiratory pathogens on contact, warms and moistens the lungs, and loosens phlegm.

Taken internally, thyme has an antimicrobial effect in the gut and is warming and stimulating to the whole digestive system. This can explain why thyme is such an important culinary herb—improving digestion and protecting from food-borne pathogens.

Topically, thyme's antimicrobial action fights infection and is strongly antifungal. Infused into apple cider vinegar, alone or with other herbs such as calendula and garlic, thyme can be a very effective remedy for athlete's foot and other fungal infections.

Recommended Dosage

Thyme is a food herb, and adding it to recipes is a great way to make it part of your daily life. For respiratory infection, thyme steams should be started at the first sign of symptoms. Even better, do steams as a preventive treatment throughout cold and flu season. Thyme can be applied topically several times a day for antimicrobial effect until the issue resolves.

Thyme steams are effective for colds and flu, but tricky for kids: The boiling water is a safety issue, and they don't like the intensity of the steam up close to their faces. When her daughter was young, Katja used blankets over a table to make a "tent" and put the pot of water to steam inside for both of them. Filling the tent with steam is more dilute and kid friendly than putting your face right over it, and Katja was there to make sure Amber didn't accidentally touch the hot pot.

Important Considerations

Thyme is very warming and may be too much for children. Sage or fennel can be substituted for internal actions and pine or peppermint for steams. Formulating thyme with gentler herbs, such as chamomile, can also help make the heat less intense.

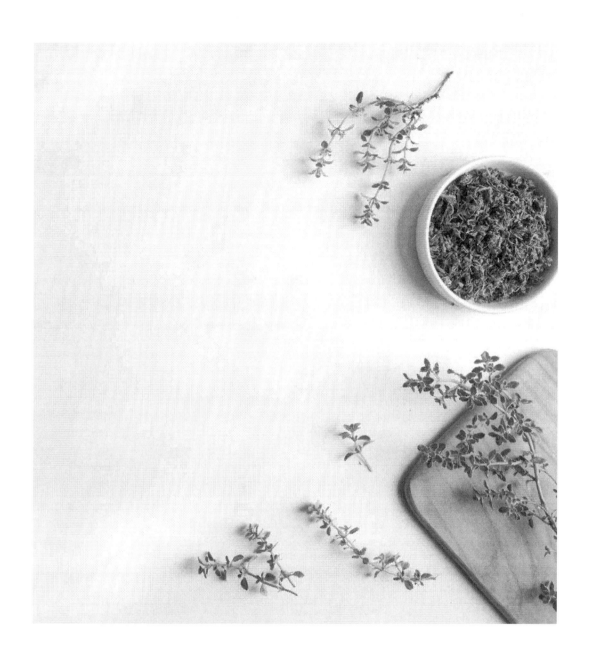

Tulsi, or Holy Basil Ocimum sanctum, tenuiflorum

Qualities: warming, drying, relaxant

Taste: aromatic, sweet, pungent, bitter

Family: Lamiaceae

Medicinal parts: leaves and flowers

Actions: adaptogen, antimicrobial, anxiolytic, aromatic, diaphoretic, diffusive, exhilarant, hepatic, hypoglycemic, immunomodulator, nervine

Common Preparations

Tulsi, also known as holy basil, can be infused into water for tea, or made as a tincture or elixir. Fresh tulsi leaves and flowers can be infused into honey.

Ideal for Addressing

- ADD/ADHD
- Anxiety
- Depression
- Fatigue
- Fever
- Food sensitivities
- Headache
- Heart palpitations
- Hypoglycemia
- Hypothyroidism
- Menopause/andropause
- PCOS
- PMS

- Seasonal depression
- Stress

Effective Applications

Tulsi has traditionally been the herb of choice for "stuck emotions," whether that's depression or PTSD or just a case of the grumpies. Recent discoveries have shown tulsi's ability to restore function to the part of the brain that processes short-term memory into long-term memory: Tulsi, literally, helps move us past difficult experiences and emotions! Tulsi is also an exhilarant, uplifting the spirit, which is a vital part of the work of releasing tension, depression, and stagnation that prevents people from successfully making lifestyle changes.

Tulsi is an *adaptogen,* meaning it helps keep hormones in check. Most people think about reproductive hormones first, but there are many hormones in the body with many different functions. Because it can help keep hormones in balance, tulsi can help with a wide variety of issues—from trouble sleeping to blood sugar regulation to menopause.

Tulsi also has a special ability to help moderate cravings, which makes it the perfect partner for people trying to reduce sugar intake, eliminate food allergies, or quit smoking or drinking.

Another of the mint family diaphoretics, tulsi is a handy helper for fever and flu. Tulsi relaxes the body and stimulates circulation, helping "sweat out" a fever.

Recommended Dosage

Tulsi makes a tasty tea you can drink all day long. It blends well with other herbs and makes a tasty elixir, too—take as needed in any stressful moment. Work with tulsi freely: This mood booster also has mineral and vitamin content.

Important Considerations

Tulsi is a safe herb for all ages, including people taking antidepressant and psychiatric medications. *However, if you take blood sugar management pharmaceuticals, monitor your glucose levels regularly because tulsi can have a significant blood sugar–lowering effect.*

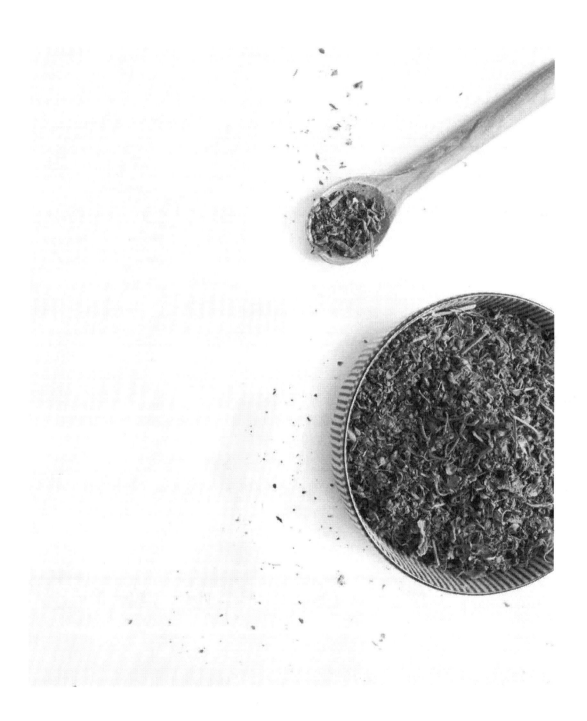

Uva-Ursi Arctostaphylos uva-ursi

Qualities: cooling, drying, tonifying

Taste: astringent, pungent

Family: Ericaceae

Medicinal parts: leaves

Actions: diuretic, respiratory astringent, topical antifungal and antimicrobial (biofilm disruptor), urinary astringent and antimicrobial, uterine astringent

Common Preparations

Uva-ursi leaves can be prepared as a tea or tincture.

Ideal for Addressing

- Abscess and gingivitis
- Athlete's foot/fungal skin infections
- BPH/prostatitis
- Edema
- Gout
- Incontinence
- Kidney stones
- Rash
- Receding gums
- UTI
- Yeast infection

Effective Applications

Taken internally, uva-ursi has particular affinity for the urinary system and pelvic floor, where its astringency supports against BPH and prostatitis, incontinence, and other prolapse issues, including edema. This astringency can also be effective topically for treating weepy rashes, abscesses, spongey and receding gums, and other issues that require draining.

Uva-ursi has a very strong biofilm-disrupting action, which is excellent for fighting infection topically and in the urinary tract. When cranberry juice isn't enough to stop a UTI, it may be because the bacteria have had enough time to band together and establish a biofilm. Uva-ursi can break up the bacteria so your immune system can fight it.

Recommended Dosage

Because it's so focused on urinary system issues, it's best to work with uva-ursi in water. For acute issues, 2 to 4 cups of tea daily is appropriate. If the flavor is too astringent, tincture can be taken instead, but in that case it's important to increase overall liquid intake for the day: Clearing kidney and urinary tract issues requires plenty of fluids. Topically, uva-ursi can be applied as a soak or compress several times daily as needed and orally as a rinse at least 3 times a day.

Important Considerations

A kidney stimulant, *uva-ursi should not be given to individuals with kidney disease*; for these individuals, use goldenrod and nettle instead. Uva-ursi is a very strong herb and should not be taken in large doses for extended periods—generally, not longer than 2 weeks at a time. For longer-term use, formulate with herbs such as goldenrod and self-heal to soften its effect. Do not blend uva-ursi with marshmallow root, as the tannins in uva-ursi will bind with the mucilagens in marshmallow, resulting in an unpleasant sludge.

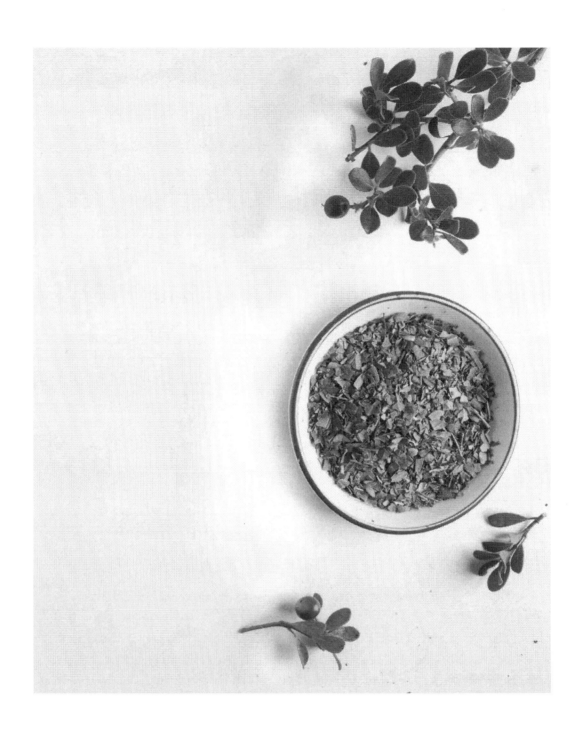

Wild Lettuce Lactuca virosa, spinosa

Qualities: cooling, drying, relaxant

Taste: bitter

Family: Asteraceae

Medicinal parts: leaves, stems, latex (sap)

Actions: anodyne, antimicrobial, antispasmodic, bitter, hepatic, hypnotic, nervine, refrigerant, sedative

Common Preparations

Wild lettuce stalks and leaves can be prepared as a tea or tincture. Wild lettuce latex can be tinctured for a stronger pain-relieving preparation.

Ideal for Addressing

* Anxiety
* Back pain
* Fever
* Headache
* Insomnia
* Muscle soreness/post-workout recovery
* Pain management

Effective Applications

A cooling and relaxing hypnotic (sleep-inducing) herb, wild lettuce is particularly appropriate when pain prevents sleep or causes agitation, anxiety, and nervousness. Even when dealing with severe pain caused by illness or injury, wild lettuce cools the sensation, removing enough pain so sleep can occur.

Wild lettuce is also a cooling bitter and very helpful for people with hot pain in the stomach—whether from physiological factors such as ulcers or heartburn or emotional factors such as high stress levels and anxiety.

Wild lettuce's pain-relieving constituents are concentrated in the plant's white, milky sap found in the stems. For this reason, including the stems in teas and tincture is important.

Recommended Dosage

Wild lettuce is bitter and is not generally enjoyable alone as tea. To work with wild lettuce on its own, tincture may be the more palatable option. Start with 1 to 3 droppersful as needed. For pain that makes it difficult to sleep, try pulse dosing 1 to 3 droppersful before bed (see Insomnia). For milder discomfort, blending wild lettuce with chamomile (and ginger, if desired) will create a much more palatable, and quite effective, tea.

Important Considerations

The latex-like sap of wild lettuce must be processed by the kidneys; *a latex tincture is not appropriate for individuals with existing kidney disease or dysfunction.* Additionally, if you have a latex allergy, there is some potential for allergic reaction to the sap of wild lettuce.

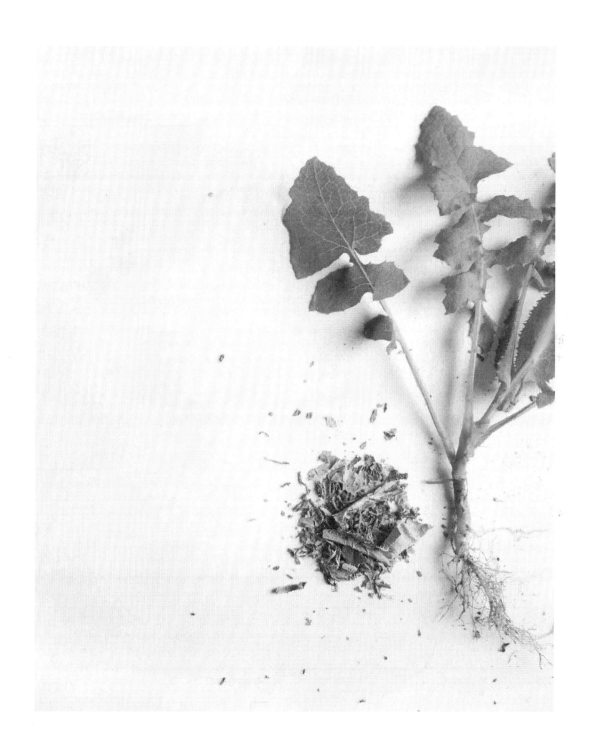

<u>Yarrow</u> Achillea millefolium

Qualities: cooling, drying, tonifying
Taste: bitter, pungent, aromatic
Family: Asteraceae
Medicinal parts: leaves and flowers
Actions: anodyne, anti-inflammatory, antimicrobial, aromatic, astringent, bitter, diffusive, diuretic, emmenagogue, hepatic, stimulant, stimulating diaphoretic, styptic

Common Preparations

Yarrow can be prepared as an infusion for tea or as a wash, compress, poultice, or soak. Yarrow can also be tinctured.

Ideal for Addressing

- Abscess and gingivitis
- Acne
- Bites and stings
- BPH/prostatitis
- Cholesterol management
- Cold and flu
- Eczema and dermatitis
- Edema
- Fever
- Food sensitivities
- Gout
- High blood pressure/hypertension
- Inflammation
- Leaky gut

- Muscle soreness/post-workout recovery
- PMS
- Rash
- Receding gums
- Stomach ulcer/gastritis
- UTI
- Varicose veins and hemorrhoids
- Wounds

Effective Applications

Topical applications of yarrow deliver an antimicrobial and astringent effect. Washes or poultices can help quite a lot with rashes, wounds, insect bites, and pimples—especially when in a wet or weepy stage.

Yarrow is a strong styptic (an agent that can stop bleeding) when applied topically, due to its tightening effect on broken blood vessels. This same effect, when applied on unbroken skin, will help drain stagnant fluids from a bruise, varicose vein, or hemorrhoid, while the anti-inflammatory constituents known as flavonoids strengthen the blood vessels and restore their integrity.

All these actions apply in the mouth, too, when yarrow is included in a mouthwash for abscess, gingivitis, or receding gums. Yarrow's astringency helps tonify lax mucous membranes in the digestive tract, too, helping restore healthy barriers that have been damaged by food allergy or leaky gut syndrome.

When taken internally, yarrow's influence is primarily over fluid movement and quality. Yarrow thins the blood slightly, lowering cholesterol levels and reducing blood pressure. Its diffusive, stimulating diaphoretic action means an improvement in blood flow from the body's core to the surface skin layers. This helps dispel a fever's heat but also provides better tissue nourishment to help the body cope with skin troubles such as eczema and dermatitis.

Yarrow acts as a moderate-strength diuretic. It can drain stagnant fluids that contribute to a sluggish period, swollen prostate, or other expressions of edema. Stimulating kidney activity and urine flow also prevents or resolves gout. Yarrow is a helpful component of formulas for treating UTI.

Like all bitter herbs, yarrow supports liver function. This improves clearance of hormones from the system and directly lessens hormonal troubles like PMS. The liver-aiding action also enhances yarrow's systemic anti-inflammatory effects and, of course, improves digestion and assimilation of nutrients from food.

Recommended Dosage

One to 3 droppersful of yarrow tincture is an effective dose and may be repeated 1 to 3 times daily. As infusion, up to a quart of yarrow tea can be taken in a day. Yarrow is safe to take long term.

Important Considerations

Yarrow has a bitter flavor when prepared on its own, so it's often best to work with it in formulas containing other, more pleasant-tasting herbs. Some people have an allergic reaction to yarrow or the whole Asteraceae family of plants. Avoid large doses during pregnancy.

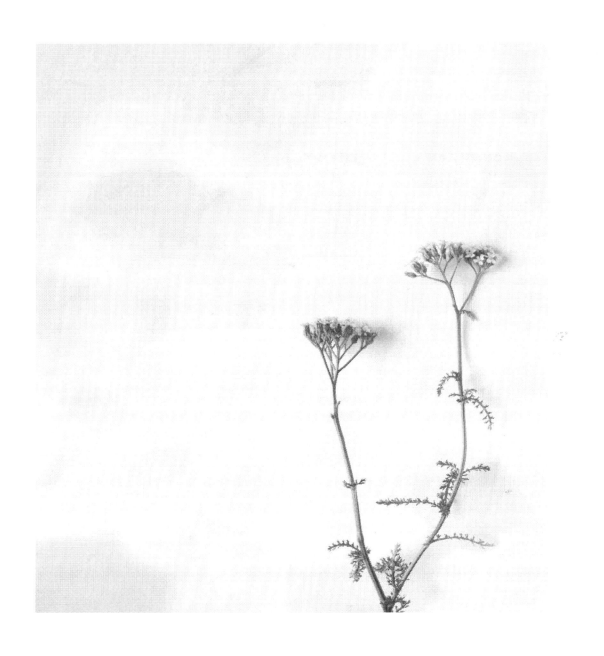

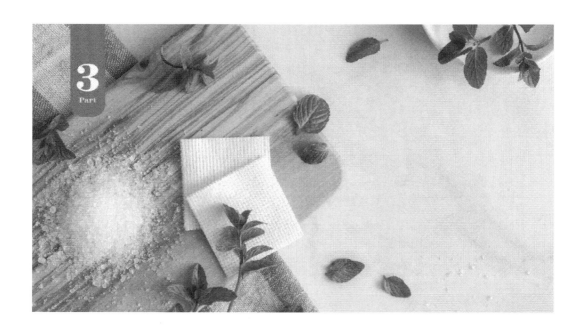

Remedies for Common Ailments

For each ailment that follows, we provide a few insights into what's going on from an herbalist's point of view. We'll note which *tissue states* are to be addressed and which *herbal actions* are needed to do so, and we'll include a list of *herbal allies*—plants that have helpful activity relevant to each ailment. Finally, we share 104 formulas for herbal preparations we use to address the ailment. Each has information about how to make and take the remedy, as well as notes about variations, optional add-ins, or potential safety concerns.

The herbal allies presented are helpful for the ailment in their own ways. They're not *exactly* interchangeable with each other, because each herb is unique, but feel free to experiment with replacing herbs that don't appeal to you (or that you don't have on hand) with others from the list of allies.

Think of each formula as a starting place, not as anything set in stone. Herbalism is as much art as it is science, and that's especially true when it comes to formulation. Individual variation is a necessary part of making good herbal remedies, so don't be afraid to experiment!

<u>Abscess and Gingivitis</u>

Relevant tissue states: heat (inflammation), dampness, laxity
Relevant herbal actions: anti-inflammatory, antimicrobial, astringent, vulnerary

Herbal Allies

- Calendula flower
- Chamomile flower
- Goldenrod leaf and flower
- Licorice root
- Meadowsweet flower
- Plantain leaf
- Rose
- Sage leaf
- Self-heal leaf and flower
- Thyme leaf
- Uva-ursi leaf
- Yarrow leaf and flower

It can be very painful to have an abscess—a fluid-filled blister or infection—in the mouth. Gingivitis is an inflammation of the gums that can lead to loose teeth. Resist the urge to poke and prod at the gums too much—if you make them bleed, bacteria can move deeper. Treat your gums gently! Antimicrobial, astringent, anti-inflammatory, and wound-healing herbs fight infection and restore healthy tissue.

HERBAL MOUTHWASH

Makes 8 fluid ounces (16 to 20 swishes)

While saltwater works well on its own, adding herbs makes it much more effective. Adjust the amounts of each herb according to taste. Swish with ¼ to ½ fluid ounce of mouthwash after brushing, and swish well, getting between the teeth and throughout the mouth, for 2 to 5 minutes.

4 fluid ounces water

1 teaspoon sea salt

1 fluid ounce tincture of uva-ursi

1 fluid ounce tincture of yarrow

½ fluid ounce tincture of calendula

½ fluid ounce tincture of plantain

½ fluid ounce tincture of self-heal

¼ fluid ounce tincture of licorice

¼ fluid ounce tincture of meadowsweet

1. In a jar with a lid, combine all the ingredients. Cover the jar, label it, and shake well. This is shelf stable.
2. Use this mouthwash every time you brush—twice a day is best.

Acne

Relevant tissue states: heat (inflammation), dampness (oily)
Relevant herbal actions: anti-inflammatory, antimicrobial, astringent, circulatory stimulant, liver stimulant, lymphatic

Herbal Allies

- Calendula flower
- Chamomile flower
- Dandelion root
- Elder
- Milk thistle seed

- Rose
- Sage leaf
- Self-heal leaf and flower
- St. John's wort leaf and flower
- Thyme leaf
- Yarrow leaf and flower

To cope with chronic skin problems, it's important to treat the issue from both the inside and the outside. Topical applications (compresses, poultices, and steams) of astringent, anti-inflammatory, and antimicrobial herbs will clear and tone the skin directly. Internal preparations (tea, tincture, capsules) of liver-stimulating, circulatory-stimulant, and lymphatic herbs support the health and nourishment of skin tissue from beneath.

SKIN TONER

Makes 12 fluid ounces (90+ applications)

The acidity and probiotics from the vinegar combine with the astringency of the witch hazel and rose to gently but effectively tonify the skin, reducing blemishes and protecting against breakouts. Be consistent; results will begin to show after a few days to a week of use. This simple skin toner is a key part of Katja's vibrant skin protocol. (Though she's 44 years old, everyone thinks she's a decade younger.) If your skin is sensitive, reduce the amount of apple cider vinegar.

4 fluid ounces apple cider vinegar (preferably raw, unfiltered)

4 fluid ounces nonalcoholic witch hazel extract

4 fluid ounces rose water, or strong, well-strained rose petal infusion

1. In a small nonreactive bowl, stir together the vinegar, witch hazel, and rose water. This mixture is shelf stable. Store in an airtight container.
2. Apply this toner once a day after washing your face. If your skin tends toward dryness, rub a few drops of oil (rosehip or olive) into the skin afterward.
3. Apply this toner a second or third time during the day if your acne is persistent, but don't scrub too hard or use harsh soaps—just rinse gently with water first.

FACIAL STEAM

Makes 2 cups dried herb mix (4 to 8 steams)

For an active breakout, especially one that is oily, a steam is a great way to effectively deliver circulation-enhancing, inflammation-reducing, and bacteria-eliminating herbal action right into the pores.

½ cup dried chamomile flower

½ cup dried sage leaf

½ cup dried thyme leaf

½ cup dried yarrow leaf and flower

½ gallon water

1. In a small bowl, stir together the chamomile, sage, thyme, and yarrow. Store in an airtight container.
2. Clean your face with gentle soap and water.
3. Make and execute an herbal steam: In a medium pot over high heat, boil the water. Place the pot on a heat-proof surface, someplace where you can sit near it, and make a tent with a blanket or towel. Add ¼ to ½ cup of the herb mixture to the water. Position your face over the steam and remain

there for 5 to 20 minutes. (Bring a tissue; the steam also clears your sinuses!)

4. Follow with spot applications of raw or herb-infused honey.

ADD/ADHD

Relevant tissue states: heat (excitation), tension

Relevant herbal actions: grounding, nervine, nutritive, relaxant, sedative

Herbal Allies

- Angelica
- Ashwagandha root
- Betony leaf and flower
- Catnip leaf and flower
- Chamomile flower
- Kelp
- Linden leaf and flower
- St. John's wort leaf and flower
- Tulsi leaf

True resolution of attention deficit and hyperactivity disorders requires significant attention to diet, sleep patterns, and lifestyle factors. For instance, a 2007 study by McCann et al., published in the *Lancet*, found that hyperactivity was strongly exacerbated by artificial colors and flavors in drinks. We have found removing food allergens and reducing sugar and caffeine intake very helpful in working with ADD and ADHD, along with adequate sleep and quiet time, and lots of physical activity. Herbs can make these transitions much easier and also markedly improve day-to-day ease in the world. We work with herbs to ground a restless mind, improve focus, and—when necessary—sedate anger and agitation.

GROUNDING TEA

Makes 2¾ cups dried herb mix (enough for 18 to 22 quarts of tea)

Betony is a standout herb for treating ADD, with its particular talent for bringing the center of consciousness into the body and the present moment. The herbal allies, catnip and chamomile, help quell anxious expressions that affect digestion —a common problem for those with ADD. If you have a dry constitution, replace the catnip with linden. Meanwhile, tulsi helps cope with the stress these disorders induce, and St. John's wort supports clearance at the liver. Drink a quart or more every day.

1 cup dried betony leaf and flower

½ cup dried catnip leaf and flower

½ cup dried chamomile flower

½ cup dried tulsi leaf

¼ cup dried St. John's wort leaf and flower (see Tip)

1. In a medium bowl, mix together all the herbs. Store in an airtight container.
2. Make a hot infusion: Prepare a kettle of boiling water. Measure 2 to 3 tablespoons of herbs per quart of water, and place in a mason jar or French press. Pour in the boiling water, cover, and steep for 20 minutes or until cool enough to drink.

TIP: Omit the St. John's wort if you are concurrently taking pharmaceuticals.

FOCUSING TINCTURE

Makes 2 fluid ounces (30 to 60 doses)

Angelica's grounding bitterness, ashwagandha's capacity to restore normal rhythms of energy and rest, betony's gentle settling-down action, and tulsi's soothing warmth help relieve moments of acute distraction. With ongoing use, it builds the ability to focus more easily and for longer periods. Take whenever a calming and centering influence is desired.

½ fluid ounce tincture of angelica

½ fluid ounce tincture of ashwagandha

½ fluid ounce tincture of betony

½ fluid ounce tincture of tulsi

1. In a small bottle, combine the tinctures. Cap the bottle and label it.
2. Take 1 to 2 droppersful at morning and noontime.

Allergies

Relevant tissue states: heat (inflammation), laxity (of the mucous membranes)

Relevant herbal actions: antihistaminic, anti-inflammatory, kidney supportive, liver stimulant

Herbal Allies

- Calendula flower
- Goldenrod leaf and flower
- Milk thistle seed
- Mullein leaf
- Nettle leaf
- Plantain leaf
- Self-heal leaf and flower

Allergic reactions to pollen, dust, or pets are primarily due to excessive histamine production, which ignites the inflammation underlying the runny nose, itchy eyes, and excessive phlegm. Histamine isn't all bad, though; it's a necessary part of sleep regulation, brain function, and even sexual response! *Antihistaminic herbs* are ideal because, while they help relieve allergy symptoms, they won't overshoot the mark and suppress histamine so much they cause adverse effects.

When trying to resolve allergies, we also must support the liver and kidneys. Among other things, the liver produces *histaminase*—an enzyme that breaks down histamine. So, when it's sluggish or overworked, histamine builds up and the inflammatory response worsens. The kidneys also help clear inflammatory instigators from the system, so giving them extra support helps reduce allergic symptoms. See also Food Sensitivities.

ALLERGY RELIEF TEA

Makes about 3 to 4 cups dried herb mix (enough for 18 to 22 quarts of tea)

Nettle and goldenrod contain the antioxidant quercetin, which, according to a 2006 study by Shaik et al., stabilizes mast cells and prevents the release of histamine. Meanwhile, mullein supports the mucous membranes in the lungs and sinuses, reducing phlegm and mucus and quelling cough. Calendula and licorice improve liver function. Feel free to add some honey to your tea—especially if it's raw, local honey! Unfiltered honey helps reduce allergic response because it contains some pollen grains. Introducing these to the body through the oral route helps it become less reactive to them when you inhale pollen in the springtime.

1 cup dried nettle leaf (see Tips)
1 cup dried goldenrod leaf and flower

½ cup dried mullein leaf

½ cup dried calendula flower

½ to 1 cup marshmallow leaf (optional)

2 to 4 tablespoons dried licorice root

1. In a medium bowl, mix together all the herbs, including the marshmallow (if using, for a dry constitution). Store in an airtight container.
2. Make a long infusion: Prepare a kettle of boiling water. Measure 2 to 3 tablespoons of herbs per quart of water and place in a mason jar or French press. Pour in the boiling water, cover, and steep for 8 hours, or overnight.
3. Drink a quart or more every day, especially in the month before and during your personal peak allergy season. The earlier you start, the less you'll suffer.

TIP: Omit the nettle leaf and increase the goldenrod if you take blood-thinning pharmaceuticals.

TIP: Want a quick fix? No time for tea? The simple combination of freeze-dried nettle leaf capsules and milk thistle seed capsules offers quick relief from allergy. Choose a high-quality brand, and take 2 of each (with plenty of water) every 4 hours.

Anxiety

Relevant tissue states: heat (excitation), tension

Relevant herbal actions: anxiolytic, nervine, relaxant, sedative

Herbal Allies

* Betony leaf and flower
* Catnip leaf and flower
* Chamomile flower
* Elderflower

- Goldenrod leaf and flower
- Linden leaf and flower
- Rose
- Tulsi leaf

Anxiety is a kind of agitation and uncomfortable excitation, so we'll work with calming, relaxing herbs to rebuild nervous system function and relaxation. Herbs for anxiety are very individual; you'll likely need to experiment with several to find the one that's most helpful for you.

Anxiety and insomnia often come together, and each worsens the other. Poor sleep stresses the body, lessening immune surveillance, detoxification, and growth and repair functions; this makes anxiety symptoms worse. See also Insomnia.

NERVINE TEA

Makes 3½ cups dried herb mix (enough for 20 to 28 quarts of tea)

Mind-calming betony and stress-melting tulsi are the best herbs we know for anxious states. This formula combines them with digestive herbs because anxiety often affects the digestive system. Elderflower helps the "heat" dissipate, and rose calms the heart.

If your anxiety manifests more strongly as digestive upset (heartburn, nausea), swap the betony and tulsi with chamomile and catnip. Consider adding goldenrod leaf and flower (¼ to ½ cup). Definitely add linden (½ to 1 cup) if you have a dry constitution or your anxiety manifests with a racing heart and high blood pressure. Drink a quart or more every day.

1 cup dried betony leaf and flower

1 cup dried tulsi leaf

½ cup dried chamomile flower

½ cup dried catnip leaf and flower

¼ cup dried elderflower

¼ cup dried rose petals

1. In a medium bowl, mix together all the herbs. Store in an airtight container.

2. Make a hot infusion: Prepare a kettle of boiling water. Measure 2 to 3 tablespoons of herbs per quart of water and place in a mason jar or French press. Pour in the boiling water, cover, and steep for 20 minutes or until cool enough to drink.

TINCTURE VARIATION: This nervine blend can also be prepared as a tincture. Using the same proportions listed (i.e., 1 *fluid ounce* tincture of betony, ½ *fluid ounce* tincture of chamomile, etc.), mix your tinctures together and bottle. Add a bit of honey to make this an elixir (see here)—that sweetness is pleasing and reassuring when we're stressed. Take 1 to 8 droppersful as needed.

JUST LINDEN

Makes 2 to 3 tablespoons dried herb yields 1 quart of tea

If your mind is spinning too much to think about which herb is right for you, and following a recipe seems too difficult, this is a time for Just Linden. Whether you take it as tea or a tincture (if you prefer, take 1 to 4 droppersful as needed), it's delicious, and very effective. Sometimes, one plant can be a complete formula all by itself!

Dried linden leaf and flower, as needed

Make a hot infusion: Prepare a kettle of boiling water. Measure 2 to 3 tablespoons of linden per quart of water and place in a mason jar or French press. Pour in the boiling water, cover, and steep for 20 minutes or until cool enough to drink.

Arthritis

Relevant tissue states: heat (inflammation), dryness or dampness (stagnation)

Relevant herbal actions: anti-inflammatory, antioxidant, demulcent, joint lubricant, nutritive, rubefacient

Herbal Allies

- Cinnamon bark
- Ginger
- Kelp
- Licorice root
- Marshmallow
- Meadowsweet flower
- Nettle leaf (its sting)
- Peppermint essential oil
- Self-heal leaf and flower
- Solomon's seal root

There are two major kinds of arthritis: osteoarthritis and rheumatoid. In osteoarthritis, pain arises due to cartilage deterioration and synovial fluid loss; it is, at root, a condition of dryness, and mainly affects elders. Rheumatoid arthritis is an autoimmune condition in which sustained inflammation causes pain and breakdown of tissue; it's strongly exacerbated by food intolerances and more often presents with stagnant fluid buildup in the joints. Both can be symptomatically addressed by many of the same herbs, but for best results we want to know whether damp or dry is the dominant tissue state.

231

If you're feeling brave, try an old reliable remedy: Sting your aching joints with nettles! Several brisk stings on the affected joints will do it. This brings fresh blood to the tissues and disperses inflammatory detritus. The stinging sensation usually fades away in 30 minutes or so, but relief from arthritic pain follows and lasts 1 day to 1 week.

JOINT SUPPORT DECOCTION

Makes 2½ cups dried herb mix (enough for 12 to 16 quarts of tea)

Kelp's nutritive values and ginger's anti-inflammatory power combine with Solomon's seal's joint support and self-heal's lymphatic stimulation. And, while unusual in a tea, at this proportion you'll hardly taste the seaweed! This is great to drink before or during yoga class or other stretching exercises. Effects may take some time to become apparent. Be patient and keep at it.

1 cup dried Solomon's seal root

⅓ cup dried ginger

⅓ cup dried meadowsweet flower

⅓ cup dried self-heal leaf and flower

¼ cup dried licorice root

¼ cup dried kelp

Cinnamon, cardamom, cloves, or allspice (optional, for flavor, and a little extra antioxidant benefit; see Tip)

1. In a medium bowl, mix together all the ingredients, including the flavoring spices (if using) as desired. Store in an airtight container.

2. Make a decoction: Measure 2 to 4 tablespoons of herbs per quart of water and place in a lidded pot over high heat. Add

the water and cover the pot. Bring to a boil, reduce the heat, and simmer for 1 hour.

3. Strain and drink.

TIP: If you opt for the cinnamon, cardamom, cloves, or allspice for flavor, add these as part of your dried mix, or prepare your tea with a pinch or two added for extra flavor depending on what you want each day. It's easy and completely up to you! Many of the same herbs used here can also be applied topically. Using both applications gives faster results than either alone. Check out Joint Liniment.

Asthma

Relevant tissue states: tension (constriction), dryness
Relevant herbal actions: anti-inflammatory, demulcent, expectorant, relaxant

Herbal Allies

- Elecampane root
- Fennel seed
- Licorice root
- Marshmallow
- Mullein leaf

Though some herbs can interrupt an acute asthma attack, they are not covered in this book. The herbs and remedies mentioned here restore lung health over time and reduce the severity of chronic asthma symptoms. To observe the effects of these remedies, do breathing exercises before and after you take the herbs. A simple exercise is square breathing: Breathe in, hold, breathe out, and hold again, counting to four during each step. Cycle through 10 times. This builds resilience in the lungs—and works even better when paired with herbs!

LUNG-STRENGTHENING TEA

Makes 2¼ cups dried herb mix (enough for 14 to 18 quarts of tea)

The herbs here relax the lungs and induce the mucous membranes to release a little more fluid, soothing the racking dry cough. They also reduce inflammation in the lungs and, if there is any mucus present, help expectorate it. Drink a quart or more every day.

1 cup dried mullein leaf

½ cup fennel seed

½ cup dried marshmallow leaf

¼ cup dried licorice root

1. In a medium bowl, mix together all the herbs. Store in an airtight container.
2. Make a hot infusion: Prepare a kettle of boiling water. Measure 2 to 3 tablespoons of herbs per quart of water and place in a mason jar or French press. Pour in the boiling water, cover, and steep for 20 minutes or until cool enough to drink.

LUNG-STRENGTHENING TINCTURE

Makes 4 fluid ounces (60 to 120 doses)

Elecampane is a strong lung stimulant; paired with relaxant mullein and soothing sweet licorice, it builds up weak lungs and protects against infection, to which asthmatics are more susceptible.

2 fluid ounces tincture of mullein

1 fluid ounce tincture of elecampane

1 fluid ounce tincture of licorice

1. In a small bottle, combine the tinctures. Cap the bottle and label it.
2. Take 1 to 2 droppersful 3 to 5 times per day.

Back Pain

Relevant tissue states: tension (spasms), heat (inflammation)
Relevant herbal actions: analgesic, anti-inflammatory, antispasmodic, relaxant

Herbal Allies

- Ginger
- Goldenrod leaf and flower
- Meadowsweet flower
- Mullein root
- Solomon's seal root
- Wild lettuce

Back pain can have many causes—injury, spasms, sciatica (nerve pain), disc problems, and so on. Long-term resolution requires figuring out what exactly is the root of the problem, but in the meantime these herbs and formulas will relieve pain and release tension, allowing you to move more freely.

SPINE'S FINE TINCTURE

Makes 4 fluid ounces (40 to 120 doses)

These warming, relaxant, analgesic herbs quell the spasms responsible for most back pain, regardless of whether the pain is acute or chronic, muscular or connective, etc. If you have infused oil made from fresh goldenrod or ginger, use it as a massage oil after you apply this formula topically. For help sleeping, take 1 to 4 droppersful of tincture of wild lettuce by mouth—this will also contribute more pain-relieving action.

1 fluid ounce tincture of Solomon's seal

1 fluid ounce tincture of ginger

½ fluid ounce tincture of goldenrod

½ fluid ounce tincture of meadowsweet

½ fluid ounce tincture of mullein root (see Tip)

½ fluid ounce tincture of St. John's wort (optional; see Tip)

1. In a small bottle, combine the tinctures. Cap the bottle and label it.

2. Take 1 to 4 droppersful by mouth 3 to 5 times per day.

3. Additionally, squirt 1 to 4 droppersful into your palm and rub it into the back muscles.

TIP: If the vertebral discs are impinged or worn away, increase the mullein root to 1 fluid ounce. It specifically supports these tissues. If sciatica or other radiating nerve pain is present, include the tincture of St. John's wort (unless you are taking pharmaceuticals). It regenerates damaged nerve tissue.

WARMING COMPRESS

Makes 1 compress

This simple application provides immediate relief.

16 fluid ounces water

½ cup dried ginger (see Tip)

¼ cup Epsom salts

1. In a small pot with a tight-fitting lid over high heat, combine all the ingredients. Cover and bring to a boil. Reduce the heat and simmer for 5 minutes. Meanwhile, fill a hot water bottle.

2. Soak a cloth in the hot tea, holding it by a dry spot and letting it cool in the air until hot but comfortable to the touch.

3. Lie down and place the wet cloth over your back. Cover with a dry cloth and lay the hot water bottle on top. Get comfortable and let it soak in for 10 to 20 minutes. You should feel warmth, relaxation, and relief from pain.

4. Repeat as often as desired.

TIP: Have pain, but no dried ginger? If all you have on hand is fresh ginger from the grocery store, you can use that, too—sliced, chopped, or grated.

Bites and Stings

Relevant tissue states: heat (inflammation)

Relevant herbal actions: anti-inflammatory, astringent, lymphatic, immune stimulant

Herbal Allies

- Peppermint leaf
- Plantain leaf
- Rose
- Self-heal leaf and flower
- Yarrow leaf and flower

Whether it's mosquitoes, black flies, or fire ants, most bug bites are fairly simple: We just need to reduce the inflammation. Bee and wasp stings are a bit more intense: Here, our goals include drawing out the venom, if possible, reducing inflammation, and helping the immune system cope with the venom that has entered the body. Watch for anaphylaxis! If someone stung or bitten is having difficulty breathing, seek help immediately.

COOLING COMPRESS

Makes 1 compress

Peppermint's menthol provides a cooling sensation to the skin, while at the same time increasing blood circulation and dispersing the irritants from the bite or sting site.

16 fluid ounces water

½ cup dried peppermint leaf

¼ cup Epsom salts

1. In a small pot with a tight-fitting lid over high heat, combine all the ingredients. Cover and bring to a boil. Remove from the heat.
2. Soak a cloth in the hot tea, holding it by a dry spot and letting it cool in the air until hot but comfortable to the touch.
3. Apply the cloth to the bite or sting.

BUG BITE RELIEF SPRAY

Makes 8 fluid ounces (number of applications varies by use)

If you regularly walk through clouds of mosquitoes or black flies or live in an area infested with chiggers, you'll want this cooling, itch-relieving spray stocked for when you come inside.

4 fluid ounces nonalcoholic witch hazel extract or apple cider vinegar

2 fluid ounces tincture of rose

1 fluid ounce tincture of self-heal

1 fluid ounce tincture of yarrow

1. In a bottle with a fine-mist sprayer top, combine all the ingredients. Cap the bottle and label it.
2. Liberally spray wherever you've been bitten.

Bloating

Relevant tissue states: dampness (stagnation)
Relevant herbal actions: carminative, lymphatic

Herbal Allies

* Angelica
* Calendula flower
* Fennel seed
* Ginger
* Peppermint leaf
* Self-heal leaf and flower

Bloating may be extremely common, but it's not insignificant! When you become bloated, it's a buildup of gas in the bowels or a flood of fluid swelling in the lymphatic vessels wrapped around the intestines. Fennel and ginger are great for reducing gas, but for fluid bloating, you'll want lymphatic drainers such as calendula or self-heal. See also Food Sensitivities.

DISPERSING INFUSION

Makes 3 to 3½ cups dried herb mix (enough for 18 to 24 quarts of tea)

This helps with bloating, no matter what kind. Feel free to adjust the proportions to your taste, and if you don't have every herb, it is still effective. Be forewarned: This will induce you to pass some gas!

1 cup dried calendula flower

1 cup dried self-heal leaf and flower

½ cup fennel seed

½ cup dried ginger

½ cup dried peppermint leaf (optional)

1. In a medium bowl, mix together all the herbs, including the peppermint (if using). Store in an airtight container.
2. Make a hot infusion: Prepare a kettle of boiling water. Measure 2 to 3 tablespoons of herbs per quart of water and place in a mason jar or French press. Pour in the boiling water, cover, and steep for 20 minutes or until cool enough to drink.
3. Drink 1 to 2 teacups after meals to prevent or dispel bloating. If this is a chronic issue, drink a quart or more every day.

DISPERSING TINCTURE

Makes 4 fluid ounces (60 to 120 doses)

A few squirts of this tincture blend will disperse gas and fluid bloating alike. Bring it with you the next time you head out for pizza or go to the local diner, and pass it around after the meal!

1 fluid ounce tincture of calendula
1 fluid ounce tincture of self-heal
1 fluid ounce tincture of fennel
½ fluid ounce tincture of ginger
½ fluid ounce tincture of angelica

1. In a small bottle, combine the tinctures. Cap the bottle and label it.
2. Take 1 to 2 droppersful as needed.

Bronchitis/Chest Cold/Pneumonia

Relevant tissue states: dampness, cold (depressed vitality)
Relevant herbal actions: antimicrobial, astringent, decongestant, diaphoretic, expectorant, pulmonary tonic

Herbal Allies

- Angelica
- Elder
- Elecampane root
- Garlic
- Ginger
- Pine
- Sage leaf
- Thyme leaf

When you have a lung infection, don't suppress the cough—it's a vital response! Our goal is to cough when it's productive, so all the irritating or infectious material is expelled as you cough up phlegm, and to reduce the amount of unproductive coughing. If you can't bring up the phlegm, you may find a simple cough developing into pneumonia because of the mucus buildup. (True pneumonia is a serious condition—seek higher care. Meanwhile, take elecampane and garlic—they're your strongest allies for this problem.)

Infection-instigated coughs are usually wet, and the herbs we discuss here assume that's the case. Refer to Cough for more help determining what kind of cough you have. The goal is to get it just a little on the moist side—nice and productive—so you can expel that phlegm.

As with any respiratory condition, an herbal steam is a great remedy all on its own, combating infection and greatly improving blood circulation—which means immune activity—in the lungs. A simple steam with thyme or sage is very good for this problem.

FIRE CIDER
Makes about 1 quart

Traditional fire cider recipes are blends of pungent and aromatic stimulating expectorants that will heat you up and help you get the gunk out. In this version, we sneak in some immune stimulants and a good source of vitamin C. *Do not consume this if you take pharmaceutical blood thinners.*

1 whole head garlic, cloves peeled and chopped

1 (2-inch) piece fresh ginger, chopped

¼ cup dried pine needles

¼ cup dried sage leaf

¼ cup dried thyme leaf

¼ cup dried elderberry

¼ cup dried rose hips

2 tablespoons dried elecampane root

2 tablespoons dried angelica root

1 quart apple cider vinegar

Honey or water, for sweetening or diluting (optional)

1. In a quart-size mason jar, combine the garlic, ginger, and remaining herbs.
2. Fill the jar with the vinegar. Cover the jar with a plastic lid, or place a sheet of wax paper under the jar lid before you screw down the ring. (The coating on the bottom of metal mason jar lids corrodes when exposed to vinegar.)
3. Let the herbs macerate in the vinegar for 2 weeks or longer.
4. Strain, bottle, and label the finished fire cider. If the vinegar is too heating to be comfortable on your stomach, add some honey (up to one-fourth the total volume), or dilute your dose with water.
5. Take a shot (about ½ fluid ounce) at the first sign of mucus buildup in the lungs, and every couple hours thereafter until symptoms resolve.

Burns and Sunburn

Relevant tissue states: heat

Relevant herbal actions: anti-inflammatory, antimicrobial, antiseptic, vulnerary

Herbal Allies

- Calendula flower
- Linden leaf and flower
- Marshmallow
- Peppermint leaf
- Plantain leaf
- Rose petals
- Self-heal leaf and flower

Immediately following a burn, run cold water over the area—the skin retains heat for much longer than you'd expect. (If blisters form in the burned area, be very gentle with them and don't break them before they naturally slough off, if you can avoid it.) Then, gently clean the wound, removing any dirt or contaminant. Apply the herbs, combining antiseptics to prevent infection with cooling, wound-healing herbs to encourage tissue regeneration.

Apply any of the herbal allies in a wash, compress, poultice, or infused honey—don't use oily preparations (like salves) on burns, because they trap the heat in the tissue.

Do not underestimate the power of a marshmallow root poultice! Simply saturate a handful of marshmallow root with enough cold water to make a gloopy mass and apply it to the burn. Cover with gauze and leave in place for 20 minutes. Repeat frequently.

BURN-HEALING HONEY

Makes about 1 pint

Honey is the single best healing agent for burns: If you have nothing but plain honey, you're still in good shape. It gets even better, though, when you infuse these healing herbs into it ahead of time.

½ cup fresh calendula flower

½ cup fresh rose petals

1 pint honey, gently warmed

1. Put the calendula and rose petals in a pint-size mason jar.
2. Fill the jar with the warm honey. Seal the jar and place it in a warm area to infuse for 1 month.
3. In a double boiler, gently warm the closed jar until the honey has a liquid consistency. Strain the infused honey into a new jar, pressing the marc against the strainer to express as much honey as you can.
4. After cooling and cleaning a burn site, apply a layer of the infused honey and cover lightly with a gauze bandage. Refresh the application at least twice a day.

SUNBURN SPRAY

Makes 8 fluid ounces

A few spritzes cool the skin and begin to reduce inflammation.

1 tablespoon dried peppermint leaf

1 tablespoon dried plantain leaf

1 tablespoon dried self-heal leaf and flower

1 tablespoon dried linden leaf and flower

1 quart boiling water

4 fluid ounces rose water

1. Make a hot infusion: In a mason jar, combine the peppermint, plantain, self-heal, and linden. Pour in the boiling water, cover, and steep for 20 minutes.
2. Move the jar to the refrigerator until it's cold.
3. Strain out 4 fluid ounces of the infusion and transfer to an 8-ounce bottle with a fine-mist sprayer top. Use the remaining infusion for compresses or a cooling drink. It will keep, refrigerated, for 3 days.
4. Add the rose water to the spray bottle. Cap the bottle and label it.
5. Apply copiously and frequently. Keep the spray refrigerated when not in use.

Cholesterol Management

Relevant tissue states: heat (inflammation)

Relevant herbal actions: anti-inflammatory, antioxidant, hepatic, hypotensive

Herbal Allies

- Cinnamon bark
- Garlic
- Ginger
- Kelp
- Linden leaf and flower
- Rose
- Yarrow leaf and flower

High cholesterol is a *symptom*, not a freestanding problem. It is an indicator that systemic inflammation is damaging the blood vessels. Many things can cause this—blood sugar dysregulation, insufficient sleep, and stress are major factors—but the biggest one of all is diet.

Herbal approaches to reducing cholesterol levels primarily rely on the antioxidant power of the plants to reduce inflammation and neutralize free radicals. Eating lots of colorful fruits and vegetables, especially berries, is also very helpful.

Garlic is one of the most well-known and extensively studied herbs for reducing inflammation in the blood vessels. Adding it to your food is a simple and effective way to lower cholesterol levels and improve other blood parameters—beneficial effects start to manifest with amounts as low as two garlic cloves per day.

ANTIOXIDANT TEA

Makes about 2 cups dried herb mix (enough for 12 to 16 quarts of tea)

Gentle linden helps soften and direct the other herbs in this blend, focusing their effects on the blood vessels to improve integrity and reduce inflammation. Drink a quart or more of this tea every day.

1 cup dried linden leaf and flower

½ cup dried rose petals, hips, or a combination

¼ cup dried cinnamon bark

¼ cup dried yarrow leaf and flower

1 tablespoon dried ginger

1. In a medium bowl, mix together all the herbs. Store in an airtight container.
2. Make a hot infusion: Prepare a kettle of boiling water. Measure 2 to 3 tablespoons of herbs per quart of water and place in a mason jar or French press. Pour in the boiling water, cover, and steep for 20 minutes or until cool enough to drink.

ROSE HIP QUICK JAM

Makes about 3 ounces (2 servings)

This simple, tasty treat is a powerhouse of vitamin C, bioflavonoids, and antioxidant goodness. Mix this into your oatmeal or other hot cereal, spread it on toast, or just eat it by the spoonful!

2 tablespoons dried rosehips

2 fluid ounces water

1 teaspoon honey

1 teaspoon powdered cinnamon

1. In a cup or small bowl, stir together the rosehips and water. Let sit for about 1 hour so the rosehips soften and absorb the water. They'll gel into a jam-like substance.
2. Stir in the honey and cinnamon.
3. Prepare fresh each day for maximum potency.

Cold and Flu

Relevant tissue states: heat (inflammatory immune response)
Relevant herbal actions: antiviral, immune stimulant

Herbal Allies

- Elder
- Garlic
- Pine
- Thyme leaf
- Yarrow leaf and flower

Antibiotic treatments don't affect viral respiratory troubles like colds and flu—they only work on bacteria. Herbs, on the other hand, offer effective assistance by supporting the body's innate healing mechanisms.

Colds and flu generally cause very similar symptoms in everyone, but for each person one or another symptom will be most acute. For details on addressing specific symptoms, see Bronchitis/Chest Cold/Pneumonia; Cough; Ear Infection/Earache; Fever; Immune Support; Sinusitis/Stuffy Nose; and Sore Throat.

ELDERBERRY SYRUP

Makes about 1 quart (20 to 60 doses)

Elderberries have an amazing specific capacity to prevent flu viruses from invading the body and replicating themselves; they also fight colds and other viruses. Take this syrup in addition to remedies for your specific symptoms—1 to 3 tablespoons 3 to 5 times per day, whenever you suspect a cold or flu is present.

3 cups fresh elderberries

6 cups water

1 cinnamon stick or 1 teaspoon powdered cinnamon

1 teaspoon powdered ginger

1 teaspoon fennel seed

1 teaspoon dried chamomile flower

2 cups honey, plus more as needed (see Tip)

1. In a medium pot over high heat, combine the berries, water, and herbs. Bring to a boil. Reduce the heat and simmer, *uncovered*, for 1 to 2 hours or until reduced by half.
2. Use a spoon to mash the berries in the pot. Stir, simmer for 15 minutes more, and strain through a wire mesh sieve or cheesecloth. Squeeze the leftover berries well to get out every last bit of fluid. You should have between 2 and 3 cups of elderberry decoction.

3. Return the elderberry decoction to the pan and place it over low heat. Add an equal amount of honey, warming it gently as you stir so it mixes thoroughly with the elderberry decoction.
4. Bottle and label the syrup. It will keep in the refrigerator for several months.

TIP: Some recipes use sugar, as this creates a shelf-stable product. We try to avoid sugar, so we use honey and keep ours refrigerated. Another alternative is to also add 2 cups of tincture (in addition to the decoction and honey) to your syrup —the alcohol content will preserve it. Tinctures of ginger, garlic, pine, yarrow, and thyme are all good options.

Constipation

Relevant tissue states: cold (stagnation), dryness, tension
Relevant herbal actions: bitter, carminative, demulcent, hepatic, laxative

Herbal Allies

* Angelica
* Dandelion root
* Ginger
* Marshmallow
* Milk thistle seed
* St. John's wort leaf and flower

Sometimes, constipation is simply a sign of dehydration—drink some water! If it's a chronic issue, it may be an indication of a food allergy or simply a sign that you're not getting sufficient fiber in your diet. A good, thick, cold infusion of marshmallow solves both problems: It rehydrates better than water alone, and it includes a lot of polysaccharides and fibers that help move stool along.

Constipation, especially when ongoing, can be traced back to sluggish liver function. Bile produced by the liver is a digestive fluid, but it also lubricates the intestines; when production is low, things can get stuck. Bitters and carminatives help spur digestive function, and liver-restorative herbs (hepatics) such as milk thistle can reestablish normal function.

BOWEL-HYDRATING INFUSION

Makes 2½ cups dried herb mix (enough for 14 to 18 quarts of tea)

A bit tastier than solo marshmallow, this is a great solution for the type of constipation that often afflicts people with dry constitutions. If you have hard-to-pass, dry, little "rabbit pellet" bowel movements, this is for you. Drink a quart or more every day.

1 cup dried linden leaf and flower

1 cup dried marshmallow root

¼ cup dried cinnamon bark

¼ cup dried licorice root

1. In a medium bowl, mix together all the herbs. Store in an airtight container.
2. Make a cold infusion: Measure 2 to 4 tablespoons of herbs per quart of water and place in a mason jar or French press. Pour in cold or room-temperature water and steep for 4 to 8 hours before straining.

BOWEL-MOTIVATING TINCTURE

Makes 4 fluid ounces (30 to 60 doses)

These bitters and carminatives will spur the bowels to movement by stimulating bile flow and intestinal peristalsis.

1½ fluid ounces tincture of dandelion root

1½ fluid ounces tincture of St. John's wort

½ fluid ounce tincture of angelica root

½ fluid ounce tincture of ginger

1. In a small bottle, combine the tinctures. Cap the bottle and label it.
2. Take 2 to 4 droppersful every 20 minutes until relief occurs.

Cough

Relevant tissue states: heat (irritation) or cold (depressed vitality), dryness or dampness

Relevant herbal actions: antitussive, astringent, decongestant, demulcent, diaphoretic, expectorant, pulmonary tonic

Herbal Allies

- Fennel seed
- Ginger
- Pine
- Marshmallow
- Mullein leaf
- Sage leaf
- Thyme leaf

For herbs to work best, we need to differentiate between a *hot, dry, irritated* cough and one that is *wet, but cold and unproductive*. When the lungs are dry, you'll have a racking, relentless cough; we use moistening herbs to correct this. Wet lungs rattle or gurgle and are most likely a response to infection. See Bronchitis/Chest Cold/Pneumonia or Cold and Flu.

LUNG-LUBRICATING TEA

Makes 2¾ cups dried herb mix (enough for 18 to 22 quarts of tea)

For dry, hot lungs, these soothing and moistening herbs bring relief from a racking, unrelenting cough.

1 cup dried marshmallow root

1 cup dried mullein leaf

½ cup fennel seed

¼ cup dried licorice root, or to taste

Honey, for extra soothing (optional)

1. In a medium bowl, mix together all the herbs. Store in an airtight container.
2. Make a cold infusion: Measure 2 to 4 tablespoons of herbs per quart of water and place in a mason jar or French press. Pour in cold or room-temperature water and steep for 4 to 8 hours.
3. Strain the liquid and drink directly, or warm, if desired.
4. Add honey (if using) for extra soothing.

ANTITUSSIVE OXYMEL

Makes about 1 quart (20 to 60 doses)

An oxymel is simply a blend of vinegar and honey, which combines the astringent and stimulating effects of the vinegar with the moistening and soothing aspects of the honey. Adding lung-specific herbs makes this a go-to for coughs of all kinds.

⅓ cup dried pine needles

⅓ cup dried sage leaf

⅓ cup dried thyme leaf

¼ cup dried ginger

1 quart apple cider vinegar

Honey, as needed for topping off the jar

1. In a quart-size mason jar, combine the herbs.
2. Fill the jar four-fifths full with vinegar; top off with honey.
3. Cover the jar and let macerate for 4 weeks.
4. Strain and bottle the oxymel. Cap the bottle and label it.
5. Take 1 to 3 tablespoons as needed.

Depression

Relevant tissue states: cold (obstruction, stagnation)

Relevant herbal actions: aromatic, exhilarant, nervine

Herbal Allies

- Ashwagandha root
- Betony leaf and flower
- Chamomile flower
- Elderflower
- Goldenrod leaf and flower
- Linden leaf and flower
- Pine
- Rose
- Self-heal leaf and flower
- St. John's wort leaf and flower
- Tulsi leaf

There is no one kind of "depression." Many things can bring it on —nutritional deficiencies, too much sedentary time, a stagnant liver, a lack of sunlight (and vitamin D), gut dysbiosis, thyroid and other endocrine disorders, situational traumas and grief . . . and each requires a slightly different strategy. That may sound complex, but, fortunately, there's a common place everyone can start—self-care. Consider these remedies as a gift to yourself, something pleasant and restorative you make time for, just as you would make time to visit a friend in need.

Peace of mind isn't a thing in the ether—we make it in our bodies from food and water, movement and air. It takes time and conscious attention. It doesn't happen all at once, but each step you take makes the next one easier. So, take the easiest step first—a cup of tea, a bit of elixir—and work up from there.

See also <u>Hypothyroidism</u>, <u>Insomnia</u>, <u>Seasonal Depression</u>, and <u>Stress</u>.

THIS IS FOR YOU

Makes up to 4¼ cups dried herb mix (enough for about 30 quarts of tea)

This tea helps bring you into a moment of relaxed, attentive presence. We've both found that it helps to practice meditation while drinking this tea. Tonglen techniques taught by Pema Chödrön are extremely helpful. You may want to look at some trees while you drink your tea; they move slowly and speak gently.

1 cup dried tulsi leaf

1 cup dried betony leaf and flower

½ cup dried chamomile flower

½ cup dried linden leaf and flower

¼ cup dried elderflower (see Tips)

¼ cup dried rose petals (see Tips)

¼ cup dried goldenrod leaf and flower (see Tips)

¼ cup dried self-heal leaf and flower

¼ cup dried St. John's wort (see Tips)

1. In a medium bowl, mix together all the herbs. Store in an airtight container.
2. Make a hot infusion: Prepare a kettle of boiling water. Measure 2 to 3 tablespoons of herbs per quart of water and place in a mason jar or French press. Pour in the boiling water, cover, and steep for 20 minutes or until cool enough to drink.
3. Pour yourself a cup of tea. Settle in somewhere and drink it. Take your time. You have time. Repeat often.

TIP: If you wish, add ¼ cup of any one of these herbs, or ¼ cup each of some of them, or ¼ cup each of all of them.

TIP: Omit the St. John's wort if you are concurrently taking pharmaceuticals.

COUNT TO SEVEN
Makes about 7 fluid ounces (50 to 90 doses)

Fortifying adaptogens and uplifting woodland herbs give you a moment to pause and a breath of energy to get through your day in a focused, calm way.

2 fluid ounces tincture of ashwagandha

2 fluid ounces tincture of tulsi

2 fluid ounces tincture of betony

1 fluid ounce tincture of pine

Touch of honey (even better if it's infused with rose)

1. In a small bottle, combine all the ingredients. Cap the bottle and label it.
2. Take 1 to 4 droppersful whenever needed. Slowly count to seven. Take a deep breath.
3. Return to the world; repeat as often as necessary.

Detox

Relevant tissue states: dampness (stagnation), heat (inflammation)
Relevant herbal actions: alterative, bitter, carminative, diaphoretic, diuretic, hepatic, lymphatic, nutritive

Herbal Allies

- Angelica
- Calendula flower
- Dandelion
- Elecampane root
- Garlic
- Ginger
- Goldenrod leaf and flower
- Kelp
- Licorice root
- Milk thistle seed
- Nettle leaf
- Plantain leaf
- St. John's wort leaf and flower
- Yarrow leaf and flower

Detoxification means making improvements in nutrition, assimilation, and all the pathways of elimination. Or, put another way, it means improving the quality of what comes in, helping the good stuff get where it needs to go, and getting rid of what's harmful or burdensome.

This is the essence of the old herbal category of *alteratives*, which were often called "blood cleansers" in summation of their observable effects: better fluid movement, tissue tone, circulation, and general vitality. Such remedies have always been given together with advice on a healthy regimen, including diet, exercise and movement, sleep habits, and various ways to train the mind.

LIVER LOVE TINCTURE

Makes 8 fluid ounces (3 to 12 weeks' supply)

The liver is the great detoxifier, responsible for more breakdown and elimination of burdensome substances in the body than any other organ. With gentle stimulating and protective effects, these herbs keep the liver humming along smoothly.

1⅓ fluid ounces tincture of plantain

1⅓ fluid ounces tincture of calendula

1⅓ fluid ounces tincture of yarrow

1 fluid ounce tincture of dandelion root

1 fluid ounce tincture of angelica root

1 fluid ounce tincture of licorice

1 fluid ounce tincture of St. John's wort (see Tip)

1. In a medium bottle, combine the tinctures. Cap the bottle and label it.
2. Take 1 to 3 droppersful 3 to 5 times per day. Be consistent and persistent! Effects will continue to accrue with weeks to months of continuous use.

TIP: Omit the St. John's wort if you are concurrently taking pharmaceuticals.

ALTERATIVE TEA

Makes up to 5 cups dried herb mix (enough for 20 to 40 quarts of tea)

When it comes to alterative herbs, this is one of the few places we might say, "The formula with the most herbs wins." Because this is taken over a long period of time, it's important to adjust it to match your personal constitution. If your constitution is hot, reduce or eliminate the angelica and ginger; if cold, increase the ginger or add 1 sliced garlic clove to each quart brewed; if dry, add ½ to 1 cup marshmallow leaf or linden; if damp, increase the nettle or dandelion leaf. (See Tip.)

1 cup dried calendula flower

1 cup dried plantain leaf

½ cup dried dandelion leaf

½ cup dried goldenrod leaf and flower

½ cup dried nettle leaf

¼ cup dried angelica root

¼ cup dried ginger

¼ cup dried kelp

¼ cup dried licorice root

¼ cup dried yarrow leaf and flower

¼ cup dried St. John's wort leaf and flower

1. In a medium bowl, mix together all the herbs. Store in an airtight container.
2. Make a long infusion: Prepare a kettle of boiling water. Measure 2 to 3 tablespoons of herbs per quart of water and place in a mason jar or French press. Pour in the boiling water, cover, and steep for 8 hours or overnight.
3. Drink a quart or more every day. Continue for several weeks to months.

TIP: Combining any of these herbs in the proportions listed will yield a drinkable tea that will support the goals of the formula. So, if you don't have or don't like a particular herb, you can leave it out without losing efficacy. Omit the St. John's wort if you are concurrently taking pharmaceuticals.

Diarrhea

Relevant tissue states: laxity (barrier compromise), dampness
Relevant herbal actions: astringent, demulcent

Herbal Allies

- Cinnamon bark
- Marshmallow
- Meadowsweet flower
- Plantain leaf
- Rose
- Self-heal leaf and flower

When the lining of the bowels loses integrity, excess fluid is lost. To counteract this directly, astringent herbs restore healthy tone to the mucous membranes, so water stays in the body where it belongs. Once this is accomplished, it's a good idea to follow up with some soothing demulcent herbs—especially if the diarrhea has been going on for a while, as that causes dehydration, which must be corrected.

ASTRINGENT FORMULA

Makes 2¼ cups dried herb mix (enough for 14 to 18 quarts of tea)

The tannins in these herbs help bind lax tissues back together so fluids stay where they belong and barriers keep their integrity. Drink a quart of tea over the course of the day.

1½ cups dried self-heal leaf and flower

½ cup dried meadowsweet flower

¼ cup rose petals

1. In a medium bowl, mix together all the herbs. Store in an airtight container.
2. Make a hot infusion: Prepare a kettle of boiling water. Measure 2 to 3 tablespoons of herbs per quart of water and place in a mason jar or French press. Pour in the boiling water, cover, and steep for 20 minutes or until cool enough to drink.

TINCTURE VARIATION: If you prefer, make a tincture blend using the same proportions: Combine 1½ fluid ounces tincture of self-heal, ½ fluid ounce tincture of meadowsweet, and ¼ fluid ounce tincture of rose petal. Take 1 to 6 droppersful every 20 minutes until relief occurs.

CINNAMON POWDER CAPSULES

Makes 20 to 24 capsules

When cinnamon is extracted into water—as an infusion or decoction—its demulcent quality is emphasized. However, if you swallow a capsule of the powder, the capsule dissolves in your GI tract and releases the dry powder, which then absorbs excess water and exerts an astringent effect on the intestinal lining. This quells diarrhea quite nicely. The Capsule Machine, a handy manual capsule-filling device, helps with this recipe quite a lot.

20 to 24 empty gelatin capsules, size "00"

2 tablespoons powdered cinnamon

1. Fill the capsules with the cinnamon powder.
2. Take 1 to 3 capsules when you have diarrhea. If relief isn't obtained within an hour, take another dose.

Dry Mouth

Relevant tissue states: dryness

Relevant herbal actions: bitter, demulcent, sialagogue

Herbal Allies

- Dandelion
- Fennel seed
- Ginger
- Licorice root
- Linden leaf and flower
- Marshmallow

Insufficient saliva isn't just a nuisance—it can lead to serious and costly dental problems. Katja once had a client with such bad dry mouth that her fillings kept popping out! Fortunately, this is an easy fix with herbs: Hydrating demulcents and saliva-stimulating bitters come quickly to the rescue.

DEMULCENT WATER

Makes 3¼ cups dried herb mix (about 1 to 2 months' supply)

Not all demulcent preparations need to be out-and-out slimy. Just a little extra viscosity in your water bottle will keep your body and mouth hydrated.

1½ cups dried marshmallow root

1 cup dried linden leaf and flower

½ cup fennel seed

¼ cup dried licorice root (optional)

1. In a medium bowl, mix together all the herbs, including the licorice root (if using). Store in an airtight container.
2. Add 1 to 2 tablespoons to your water bottle at the beginning of the day. They'll infuse and exude their demulcency slowly over the course of several hours.

3. Leave the herbs in there when you refill your water bottle; they'll be good all day.
4. Discard the herbs at the end of the day and start over in the morning.

Ear Infection/Earache

Relevant tissue states: heat (inflammation)
Relevant herbal actions: antimicrobial, immune stimulant

Herbal Allies

* Garlic/onion
* Mullein flower

The pain of an earache is due to inflammation, and although that means your body is working to fight the infection, the fluid buildup is painful. Recurring ear infections lead us to suspect food sensitivities, especially in children. Let's help the body along with some herbal support. Both these remedies are topical; for internal support options, see also Immune Support and Cold and Flu.

THE "ONION TRICK"

Makes 4 to 8 steams (both ears)

Essentially, this is an "ear steam." The onion's sulfur is carried into the ear in the steam and fights the infection, either by killing microbes directly or stimulating a stronger immune response. Also, the heat is soothing—sounds simple, but it really matters.

This is the first herbal medicine Katja learned, while living as a university student in Russia. Katja has always been prone to severe and chronic ear infections, but once she learned this trick, they became quite easy to manage!

Olive oil, for lightly coating the pan

1 onion (red or yellow), cut into ¾-inch-thick flat slices (do not separate the rings)

1. In a medium skillet over high heat, heat just a bit of oil to coat the bottom of the pan.
2. Add 2 onion slices, flat-side down, and sauté lightly for 1 to 3 minutes until warm and translucent (not caramelized, just hot all the way through).
3. Wrap the onion slices in clean, soft cloths and lie down with a wrapped onion on each ear, like heating pads. Rest for about 10 minutes until they're not hot anymore, and let it work.
4. Always steam both ears; repeat as often as necessary.

TIP: If you have garlic but not onion, peel and chop the garlic a bit, sauté lightly, and pile it into a mound. Wrap in a cloth and steam as indicated.

EAR OIL

Yield varies

Garlic can be infused into oil very rapidly, so you can make it on demand, whereas mullein requires advance preparation. Mullein has a cooling rather than warming effect and is preferred when the earache is not relieved by heat, but rather worsened by it.

FOR GARLIC OIL

4 garlic cloves, peeled and chopped

¼ cup oil (olive, grapeseed, etc.)

1 mugful boiling water

FOR MULLEIN OIL

4-ounce mason jar filled with fresh mullein flowers (see Tip)

2 to 3 fluid ounces oil (olive, grapeseed, etc.), enough to fill the space in the jar

TO MAKE GARLIC OIL

1. In a small dish, combine the garlic and oil.
2. Place the dish on top of the mug of boiling water to warm the oil. Let sit for 30 minutes, then strain out the garlic.
3. Using a dropper, put 2 to 4 drops of oil in one ear as you lay your head down for 5 minutes, allowing it to settle. Switch and treat the other side.

TO MAKE MULLEIN FLOWER OIL

1. Make a fresh mullein flower–infused oil as usual (see here for complete instructions); strain.
2. Using a dropper, put 2 to 4 drops of oil in one ear as you lay your head down for 5 minutes, allowing it to settle. Switch and treat the other side.

TIP: To gather mullein flowers, you either need many mulleins or a lot of patience: On each plant, only a couple of flowers usually emerge each day. Fortunately, you don't need to make very much infused oil, as you only use a few drops each time. Mullein oil can also sometimes be purchased at your local health food store or online.

Eczema and Dermatitis

Relevant tissue states: heat (inflammation), dryness (dampness if weepy)

Relevant herbal actions: adrenal supportive, alterative, lymphatic, mucous membrane tonic

Herbal Allies

- Calendula flower

- Chamomile flower
- Kelp
- Licorice root
- Marshmallow
- Plantain leaf
- Rose
- Self-heal leaf and flower
- Yarrow leaf and flower

Eczema, a.k.a. atopic dermatitis, is a chronic inflammatory skin condition. It's primarily a condition of dryness, though sometimes the lesions are weepy. Resolving eczema outbreaks involves quelling itching, calming irritation, drying out weeping sores (if present), and restoring healthy skin tone. Most cases of eczema are tied to some sort of food allergy, so it's worth investigating that idea if you have chronic eczema.

LICORICE LOTION

Makes 1½ cups (1 to 4 weeks' supply)

Licorice is good for inflammation and dryness. Simple heat-infused dried licorice oil works well on eczema, but a lotion made with that oil is even better.

¼ cup dried licorice root

6 fluid ounces olive oil

1 ounce beeswax, chopped or grated

6 fluid ounces rose water

1. Preheat the oven to 180°F.
2. In a small oven-safe container, combine the licorice and olive oil; ideally, the root pieces should be submerged. Place in the oven for 8 hours.

3. Strain and reserve the oil.

4. Melt the wax into the licorice oil, making a salve (see <u>here</u> for complete instructions).

5. Use this salve, together with the rose water, to make a lotion (see <u>here</u> for complete instructions).

6. Bottle the lotion. Cap the bottle and label it, including *Shake well before each use*.

7. Apply to the affected area 3 to 5 times daily.

TIP: If your eczema is particularly dry, you might also apply some soft calendula and plantain salve. Make a salve as instructed <u>here</u>, but use less beeswax to make it on the soft side, more like ointment. You can leave this as is, or make it into lotion. Apply a thin layer when the eczema patches are dry, 2 to 4 times per day.

Edema

Relevant tissue states: dampness, laxity

Relevant herbal actions: astringent, circulatory stimulant, dispersive, diuretic, hepatic, lymphatic

Herbal Allies

- Calendula flower
- Dandelion
- Ginger (especially fresh)
- Rose
- Sage leaf
- Self-heal leaf and flower
- Uva-ursi leaf
- Yarrow leaf and flower

Edema is a classic problem of stagnation—stuck flow, blockage and swelling, spongy tissue quality. In time, this may lead to heat from the "stuckness," which then rises in the body—so belly edema may produce headaches, or swollen ankles may lead to inflamed hips. With herbs, we'll drain the stuck fluids and tonify the lax, boggy tissues.

FLUID MOVEMENT TINCTURE

Makes 4 fluid ounces (60 to 120 doses)

Let's get those fluids dispersed throughout the body, instead of all pooled in one place. Circulatory stimulants and lymphatics together do the job.

1¼ fluid ounces tincture of yarrow

1 fluid ounce tincture of calendula

1 fluid ounce tincture of self-heal

¾ fluid ounce tincture of ginger (ideally made with fresh root)

1. In a small bottle, combine the tinctures. Cap the bottle and label it.
2. Take 1 to 2 droppersful 3 to 5 times per day.

DRAINING TEA

Makes 5 cups dried herb mix (enough for 24 to 34 quarts of tea)

This drying blend will get the lymph flowing and the kidneys filtering. Drink a quart or more every day, and add ginger, peppermint, or rose hips for a pleasant flavor, if you like.

1 cup dried calendula flower

1 cup dried dandelion leaf (see Tip)

1 cup dried nettle leaf (see Tip)

267

½ cup dried sage leaf

½ cup dried self-heal leaf and flower

½ cup dried yarrow leaf and flower

½ cup dried uva-ursi leaf

1. In a large bowl, mix together all the herbs. Store in an airtight container.
2. Make a hot infusion: Prepare a kettle of boiling water. Measure 2 to 3 tablespoons of herbs per quart of water and place in a mason jar or French press. Pour in the boiling water, cover, and steep for 20 minutes or until cool enough to drink.

TIP: If you take pharmaceutical blood thinners, reduce the dandelion and nettle to ¼ cup each.

Endometriosis

Relevant tissue states: dampness (stagnation), heat (inflammation)
Relevant herbal actions: adaptogen, alterative, circulatory stimulant, diuretic, hepatic, lymphatic, nutritive, uterine astringent

Herbal Allies

- Angelica
- Ashwagandha root
- Calendula flower
- Dandelion
- Ginger
- Goldenrod leaf and flower
- Licorice root
- Milk thistle seed
- Nettle leaf
- Self-heal leaf and flower
- St. John's wort leaf and flower

- Tulsi leaf

When tissue that should be lining the uterus is growing elsewhere in the abdominal cavity, it leads to this painful condition. Endometriosis worsens as you go through your menses, because the misplaced tissue is still "trying to shed" as if it were part of the normal period. Restoring hormonal balance, improving pelvic circulation, and reducing inflammation systemically will mitigate endometriosis symptoms.

In our practice, we've had very good success seeing clients turn endometriosis around. In the most successful cases, elimination of gluten, dairy, soy, sugar, and caffeine made an enormous difference, along with Nettle and Friends Tea. If it seems like a lot, start with whichever action seems easiest, and progress from there!

NETTLE AND FRIENDS TEA

Makes 3½ cups dried herb mix (enough for 20 to 28 quarts of tea)

This is one variant of a blend we turn to for a wide array of problems. The nettle, dandelion, and licorice are at the core, with their nutritive and anti-inflammatory virtues; the other herbs play supporting roles. In this case, the diuretic goldenrod and lymphatic self-heal help drain stagnant fluids that increase pressure and make endometriosis pain worse. Drink a quart or more every day.

1 cup dried nettle leaf

1 cup dried dandelion leaf

½ cup dried goldenrod leaf and flower

½ cup dried self-heal leaf and flower

¼ cup dried licorice root

¼ cup dried St. John's wort leaf and flower (see Tip)

1. In a medium bowl, mix together all the herbs. Store in an airtight container.
2. Make a long infusion: Prepare a kettle of boiling water. Measure 2 to 3 tablespoons of herbs per quart of water and place in a mason jar or French press. Pour in the boiling water, cover, and steep for 8 hours, or overnight.

TIP: Omit the St. John's wort if you are concurrently taking pharmaceuticals. If taking pharmaceutical blood thinners, prepare this as a tincture instead (see here). If taking thyroid medications, wait 2 hours after taking them before consuming this infusion.

ENDOCRINE ELIXIR

Makes 5 fluid ounces (75 to 150 doses)

This elixir brings together adaptogens and pelvic circulatory stimulants to support the health of the pelvic organs.

1½ fluid ounces tincture of ashwagandha

1½ fluid ounces tincture of tulsi

¾ fluid ounce tincture of angelica

¾ fluid ounce tincture of ginger

½ fluid ounce tincture of licorice (optional)

Touch of honey

1. In a small bottle, combine the tinctures and honey. Cap the bottle and label it.
2. Take 1 to 2 droppersful 3 to 5 times per day.

Fatigue

Relevant tissue states: cold (depletion, depression, exhaustion)

Relevant herbal actions: adaptogen, exhilarant, stimulant

Herbal Allies

- Angelica
- Ashwagandha root
- Licorice root
- Tulsi leaf

Fatigue is an indication that something is impairing recovery. Most of the time, it's simply a lack of sleep. (Believe it or not, healthy adults need 8 to 10 hours of sleep a night—every night —and most Americans only get 6 on weekdays, 8 on weekends!) Even if your fatigue is not immediately relieved by a good night's sleep, it's still important to prioritize sleep. While there can be other factors in play (malnutrition, chronic illness, stress, pharmaceutical side effects, etc.), sleep is irreplaceable.

To counter fatigue, Ryn likes to emphasize the importance of movement for building energy. A little bit of motion can grow into greater kinetic energy if you cultivate it, gently and consistently. Tai chi and qigong are excellent for this.

While you're working on that, we'll draw on the talents of our adaptogens and uplifting, stimulating herbs to help break through the fog and push forward.

See also <u>Depression</u>, <u>Hypothyroidism</u>, <u>Insomnia</u>, and <u>Stress</u>.

ADD APT AID

Makes 3 fluid ounces (45 to 90 doses)

This reliable formula has garnered much praise from our clients over the years; we consider it extremely reliable for fatigue, stress, and other states of depletion.

1 fluid ounce tincture of licorice

1 fluid ounce tincture of ashwagandha

1 fluid ounce tincture of tulsi

1. In a small bottle, combine the tinctures. Cap the bottle and label it.
2. Take 1 to 2 droppersful, at morning and noontime. Feel free to take additional doses whenever you need a boost.

MORALE MORSELS

Makes about 24 pieces

These tasty, restorative treats are a good way to get a substantial dose of beneficial herbs. This format is particularly useful because it provides the full complement of plant compounds instead of just those that are water soluble or alcohol soluble, as happens with a tea or tincture.

¼ cup powdered ashwagandha root

¼ cup powdered tulsi leaf

¼ cup powdered milk thistle seed

¼ cup powdered nettle leaf

3 tablespoons powdered licorice root

¾ cup nut butter

½ cup honey

Unsweetened shredded coconut, cocoa powder, powdered cinnamon, powdered ginger, cayenne, or whatever seems tasty to you, for coating

1. In a large bowl, blend the powders together.
2. Add the nut butter and honey. Stir to form a thick "dough."
3. Roll the dough into balls about the size of a walnut (1 inch).
4. Roll the balls in your coating of choice.
5. Eat 1 to 4 per day.

Fever

Relevant tissue states: heat, dryness (dehydration)
Relevant herbal actions: diaphoretic, refrigerant

Herbal Allies

- Angelica
- Catnip leaf and flower
- Elderflower
- Garlic
- Ginger
- Peppermint leaf
- Sage leaf
- Thyme leaf
- Tulsi leaf
- Wild lettuce
- Yarrow leaf and flower

Fever is your friend: It's a vitally important immune response—and herbalists aren't the only ones saying so! The American Academy of Pediatrics released a clinical report in 2011 that stated: "It should be emphasized that fever is not an illness but is, in fact, a physiologic mechanism that has beneficial effects in fighting infection." So, don't give in to fever phobia—help your body do its work.

Stay hydrated! Almost all serious problems associated with fever come not from the fever itself but from runaway dehydration. If a person is too nauseous to keep down fluids, sitting in a warm bath is a good way to rehydrate.

Finally, remember that temperatures are relative to individuals. Children run hot, elders run cool, and constitution influences your baseline body temperature. A limp and

273

unresponsive person at 99°F is in more trouble than an active, alert person at 101°F. So, always look at the *person* more closely than the thermometer.

FEVER-MAKING TEA

Makes 3 cups dried herb mix (enough for 18 to 24 quarts of tea)

Often we want to help fever come on strong, with the help of our stimulating diaphoretics. These will help a fever be more productive, and they can also help the fever be more bearable because they cause the body to sweat. Drink a big mug of this tea whenever a fever is low and lingering and you want to boost it into an effective heat.

1 cup dried tulsi leaf

½ cup dried sage leaf

½ cup dried thyme leaf

½ cup dried yarrow leaf and flower

¼ cup dried angelica root

¼ cup dried ginger

1 garlic clove, sliced, for a real kick (optional)

1. In a medium bowl, mix together all the herbs. Store in an airtight container.
2. Make a hot infusion: Prepare a kettle of boiling water. Measure 2 to 3 tablespoons of herbs per quart of water and place in a mason jar or French press. Add the garlic (if using). Pour in the boiling water, cover, and steep for 20 minutes. For best effect, reheat before drinking and drink very hot.

FEVER-BREAKING TEA

Makes 1¾ cups dried herb mix (enough for 14 to 24 pints of tea)

If the fever is too hot to tolerate, these relaxing diaphoretics and refrigerants will relieve tension and release the heat without stimulating more fire. The wild lettuce in the mix will make you sleepy, which is good—sleep is your best healing mechanism. Go to bed!

½ cup dried catnip leaf and flower

½ cup dried elderflower

½ cup dried peppermint leaf

¼ cup dried wild lettuce leaf and stalk

1 pint boiling water

1. In a medium bowl, mix together all the herbs. Store in an airtight container.
2. Make a hot infusion: Measure 1 to 2 tablespoons of herbs and place in a pint-size mason jar. Pour in the boiling water, cover, and steep for 20 minutes or until cool. Drink this tea slightly cooler than usual.
3. Sip on a mugful when you want to reduce a fever.

Food Sensitivities

Relevant tissue states: heat (inflammation), laxity (barrier compromise)

Relevant herbal actions: bitter, carminative, demulcent, hepatic, nervine, nutritive, relaxant, vulnerary

Herbal Allies

- Calendula flower
- Catnip leaf and flower
- Chamomile flower

- Dandelion
- Fennel seed
- Ginger
- Kelp
- Licorice root
- Marshmallow
- Meadowsweet flower
- Plantain leaf
- Self-heal leaf and flower
- St. John's wort leaf and flower
- Tulsi leaf
- Yarrow leaf and flower

Food sensitivities are extremely common and run the gamut from mild to life-threateningly severe. They cause all manner of gastrointestinal upsets—heartburn, IBS, bloating, and more—but can also contribute to systemic inflammation, neurological problems, and autoimmunity.

In our opinion, everyone should periodically assess for sensitivity to a few common foods: Gluten, dairy, soy, corn, eggs, and nightshades (potatoes, tomatoes, peppers, eggplant, etc.) are all common culprits. A 30-day elimination period similar to what's described on Whole30.com, during which you avoid the suspect food entirely and track the severity of your symptoms, is the best way to identify if you have a sensitivity to a particular food.

Once your individual trigger foods are identified and eliminated from your diet, there's still some cleanup and reset work to do—that's where herbs really shine. A cup or two of herb-infused broth and a quart of gut-healing infusion in a day will have you feeling like a new person in no time.

GUT-HEAL TEA

Makes 4⅓ cups dried herb mix (enough for 20 to 40 quarts of tea)

This blend of digestive herbs combines all the actions needed to restore healthy function to the stomach, intestines, and liver. It is the single most-frequently recommended formula in our practice and is open to a wide degree of individual customization: If you have lots of gut cramping, add more chamomile and fennel. If you're constitutionally dry, add more marshmallow. If you run very hot, omit the ginger. If there's an herb you don't like, just leave it out, and if there's one you particularly love, add more! Drink a quart or more every day.

½ cup dried calendula flower

½ cup dried plantain leaf

½ cup dried chamomile flower

½ cup dried tulsi leaf

⅓ cup dried catnip leaf and flower

⅓ cup fennel seed

⅓ cup dried peppermint leaf

⅓ cup dried marshmallow leaf

¼ cup dried ginger

¼ cup dried licorice root

¼ cup dried yarrow leaf and flower

¼ cup dried St. John's wort leaf and flower (see Tip)

1. In a large bowl, mix together all the herbs. Store in an airtight container.

2. Make a hot infusion: Prepare a kettle of boiling water. Measure 2 to 3 tablespoons of herbs per quart of water and

place in a mason jar or French press. Pour in the boiling water, cover, and steep for 20 minutes or until cool enough to drink.

TIP: Omit the St. John's wort if you are concurrently taking pharmaceuticals.

BUILD-UP BROTH
Makes about 3 quarts

Bone broth is very healing to the gut, especially when the bones have bits of collagen (gristle) attached. The amino acids in these parts help restore intestinal integrity, which is compromised by the food allergy reaction. Adding herbs enhances these healing and anti-inflammatory activities. If you feel particularly awful, forego solid food for a day and just have lots of broth!

One more reason to get in the bone broth habit: Broth made from bones with collagenous tissue still attached is rich in glucosamine and chondroitin. These nutrients are utilized by the body to rebuild healthy joints and connective tissues. You can buy glucosamine and chondroitin as supplements, but bone broth is a cheaper source and has so many other additional benefits!

1 cup dried calendula flower

¼ cup dried dandelion root

¼ cup fennel seed

¼ cup dried ginger

¼ cup dried kelp

Bones (such as from 1 rotisserie chicken; 6 pork chop bones; 1 lamb or beef shank; or the bones, head, and tail from 2 medium fish—really, any bones will do . . .)

3 quarts water, plus more as needed

1 tablespoon apple cider vinegar

Oyster, shiitake, or maitake mushrooms, for their nutritive and healing properties (optional)

Salt

Freshly ground black pepper

1. In a large pot over high heat, combine the herbs, bones, water, vinegar, and mushrooms (if using). Season with salt and pepper. Bring to a boil. Sustain boiling for 4 to 8 hours. Check often and add enough water to replace what has boiled away.
2. Strain the liquid and reserve. Compost the bones and herb marc, if desired.
3. Drink a mug of warm broth 2 to 3 times per day.

Hangover

Relevant tissue states: heat (inflammation), dryness (dehydration), laxity (barrier compromise)

Relevant herbal actions: anodyne, antiemetic, anti-inflammatory, relaxant

Herbal Allies

- Betony leaf and flower
- Chamomile flower
- Ginger
- Linden leaf and flower
- Licorice root
- Marshmallow
- Milk thistle seed
- Plantain leaf
- Self-heal leaf and flower
- St. John's wort leaf and flower

Our number-one hangover preventive and simplest remedy is milk thistle capsules. Milk thistle is one of the few herbs that are very effective in capsule form, and almost all commercially available brands are good quality. The best strategy is to take 2 capsules with a big glass of water before you start drinking, another 2 before bed, and 2 more in the morning. Sometimes this will prevent you from getting a hangover at all! See also Detox, Headache, and Nausea.

EASE INFUSION

Makes about 3¼ cups dried herb mix (enough for 20 to 28 quarts of tea)

This gentle tea calms the most common hangover symptoms and helps with rehydration to boot. Best to mix it up *before* the big party, so it'll be ready when you need it. Drink a quart or more, *slowly*, over the course of the day.

½ cup dried betony leaf and flower

½ cup dried plantain leaf

½ cup dried calendula flower

½ cup dried chamomile flower

⅓ cup dried linden leaf and flower

⅓ cup dried marshmallow leaf

⅓ cup dried self-heal leaf and flower

1 tablespoon dried licorice root

1 tablespoon dried ginger

¼ cup dried St. John's wort leaf and flower (see Tip)

1. In a medium bowl, mix together all the herbs. Store in an airtight container.
2. Make a hot infusion: Prepare a kettle of boiling water. Measure 2 to 3 tablespoons of herbs per quart of water and

place in a mason jar or French press. Pour in the boiling water, cover, and steep for 20 minutes or until cool enough to drink.

TIP: Omit the St. John's wort if you are concurrently taking pharmaceuticals.

Headache

Relevant tissue states: heat or cold, damp or dry, tense or lax
Relevant herbal actions: anodyne, anti-inflammatory, astringent, circulatory stimulant, relaxant

Herbal Allies

- Betony leaf and flower
- Chamomile flower
- Ginger
- Linden leaf and flower
- Marshmallow
- Meadowsweet flower
- Sage leaf
- Tulsi leaf
- Wild lettuce

Headaches arise from a variety of imbalances. Some are simple one-off causes—dehydration, sleep debt, dietary excesses, alcohol, caffeine, medications. For those, you want quick pain relief while you supply what's missing or simply wait for the body to recover. (When unsure of where to start, turn to betony.)

For long-term relief, it's important to identify your individual triggers, as well as the underlying patterns that contribute to your pain; this takes some experimentation. These two herbal remedies are designed to address the most common types of headaches we see, but try different combinations of herbs to refine the remedy and make it as personal as possible. If you have recurrent headaches and find this helps, drink a quart or more every day as a preventive.

COOLING HEADACHE TEA

Makes 3¼ cups dried herb mix (enough for 22 to 28 quarts of tea)

If a headache makes you turn red-faced, and the pain feels hot, sharp, and very sensitive to the touch, this is for you. This kind of headache often results from tension, stress or anxiety, sinus congestion, or direct nerve pain. These herbs cool, relax (be aware the wild lettuce may make you sleepy), and drain.

1 cup dried betony leaf and flower

1 cup dried meadowsweet flower

½ cup dried linden leaf and flower

½ cup dried marshmallow leaf

¼ cup dried wild lettuce leaf and stalk

1. In a medium bowl, mix together all the herbs. Store in an airtight container.
2. Make a hot infusion: Prepare a kettle of boiling water. Measure 2 to 3 tablespoons of herbs per quart of water and place in a mason jar or French press. Pour in the boiling water, cover, and steep for 30 to 40 minutes. Drink warm or cool. One cup of this tea should begin to give some relief.

WARMING HEADACHE TEA

Makes 3¼ cups dried herb mix (enough for 22 to 28 quarts of tea)

If, when your headaches strike, you have a pale face and the pain feels cold, dull, and broad, try this blend. This type of headache is often caused by hypothyroidism, liver congestion, and circulatory stagnation. These herbs warm, gently astringe, and improve circulation. (If caffeine usually works as a headache remedy for you, try this.) If you have recurrent headaches and find this helps, drink a quart or more every day as a preventive.

1 cup dried betony leaf and flower

1 cup dried tulsi leaf

½ cup dried chamomile flower

½ cup dried sage leaf

¼ cup dried ginger

1. In a medium bowl, mix together all the herbs. Store in an airtight container.
2. Make a hot infusion: Prepare a kettle of boiling water. Measure 2 to 3 tablespoons of herbs per quart of water and place in a mason jar or French press. Pour in the boiling water, cover, and steep for 30 to 40 minutes. Drink warm to hot. One cup of this tea should begin to give some relief.

Heartburn/Reflux/ GERD

Relevant tissue states: heat (inflammation), laxity

Relevant herbal actions: bitter, carminative, demulcent, vulnerary

Herbal Allies
- Catnip leaf and flower
- Chamomile flower
- Dandelion root
- Fennel seed
- Kelp

- Licorice root
- Linden leaf and flower
- Marshmallow
- Meadowsweet flower
- Self-heal leaf and flower
- St. John's wort leaf and flower

Contrary to what you might expect, heartburn is most often caused by low levels of stomach acid. When stomach acid is low, it causes a chain of problems in the digestive system that ultimately increase upward-moving pressure in the abdomen. This weakens the "trapdoor" between the stomach and the esophagus—when that's compromised, acid is more likely to splash up through and irritate the unprotected tissue there.

Reducing stomach acid production (with antacids or acid-blocking pharmaceuticals) temporarily relieves pain, but makes the underlying problem worse. To address heartburn, first we have to heal existing damage in the esophagus or stomach (inflammation and ulcers). Then we can work to restore normal acid levels to prevent recurrence.

That stomach-esophagus "trapdoor" (the lower esophageal sphincter, LES) can also be compromised by poor alignment and stress. When in a state of stress, saliva production decreases and digestive movement is inhibited. A rest-and-digest state of mind is required to retain the proper resting tone of the LES. This starts by being present with your food—slow down, chew thoroughly, take your time.

See also Stress and Stomach Ulcer/Gastritis and H. pylori Overgrowth.

MARSHMALLOW INFUSION
Makes 1 quart

If you have active heartburn, the first thing you need is a good cold infusion of marshmallow root. Keep this on hand for when there's an attack and to heal the damaged tissue in the esophagus. When heartburn happens, just sip on this slowly and you'll feel relief in no time.

2 to 4 tablespoons dried marshmallow root

In a quart-size mason jar, combine the marshmallow with enough cold or room-temperature water to fill the jar. Cover and steep for 4 to 8 hours. Keep refrigerated, where each batch will last for 2 to 3 days.

BITTERS BLEND

Makes 3½ fluid ounces (30 to 60 doses)

To restore normal stomach acid levels and reduce the conditions for heartburn to develop, take these drops before every meal.

1 fluid ounce tincture of dandelion root

½ fluid ounce tincture of catnip

½ fluid ounce tincture of chamomile

⅓ fluid ounce tincture of fennel

⅓ fluid ounce tincture of meadowsweet

⅓ fluid ounce tincture of self-heal

½ fluid ounce tincture of St. John's wort (see Tip)

1. In a small bottle, combine the tinctures. Cap the bottle and label it.
2. Take ½ to 1 dropperful 10 minutes before eating.

TIP: Omit the St. John's wort if you are concurrently taking pharmaceuticals.

Heart Palpitations

Relevant tissue states: tension (spasm)
Relevant herbal actions: nervine, relaxant

Herbal Allies

- Betony leaf and flower
- Chamomile flower
- Ginger
- Kelp
- Linden leaf and flower
- Rose
- Tulsi leaf

Infrequent, transient chest pains can be attributed to stress or even too much caffeine, but if it happens too frequently it can be a sign of more serious heart problems. Meditation and deep breathing exercises can be particularly helpful for interrupting stressful moments and unwinding the tension that is central to this symptom. Relaxant herbs can be taken preventatively as well as in the moment. See also Stress.

WHOLE HEART TEA

Makes 3½ cups dried herb mix (enough for 20 to 26 quarts of tea)

This is a tea to drink habitually—a quart or more every day—for anyone with recurrent cardiovascular tension. Over time, it will reduce the frequency and severity of symptoms.

1 cup dried linden leaf and flower
1 cup dried betony leaf and flower
½ cup dried rose petals

½ cup dried tulsi leaf

½ cup dried chamomile flower

1. In a small bowl, mix together all the herbs. Store in an airtight container.
2. Make a hot infusion: Prepare a kettle of boiling water. Measure 2 to 3 tablespoons of herbs per quart of water and place in a mason jar or French press. Pour in the boiling water, cover, and steep for 20 minutes or until cool enough to drink.

CALM HEART ELIXIR

Makes 4 fluid ounces (60 to 120 doses)

This remedy can be taken when angina (chest pain) strikes, and it can swiftly relieve both physical and mental tension.

1 fluid ounce tincture of betony

1 fluid ounce tincture of rose petals

1 fluid ounce tincture of tulsi

⅓ fluid ounce tincture of chamomile

⅓ fluid ounce tincture of linden

⅓ fluid ounce honey

1. In a small bottle, combine the tinctures and the honey. Cap the bottle and label it.
2. Take 1 to 2 droppersful 3 to 5 times per day, or more frequently as needed whenever a heart-soothing influence is required.

Herpes/Cold Sores/Chickenpox

Relevant tissue states: heat (inflammation)

Relevant herbal actions: immune stimulant, lymphatic, vulnerary

Herbal Allies

- Calendula flower
- Chamomile flower
- Linden leaf and flower
- Plantain leaf
- Self-heal leaf and flower
- St. John's wort leaf and flower
- Thyme leaf

These common viruses are part of the same family, and the same herbs are effective for each. Together with these herbs, it will make a *major* difference in outbreak frequency and severity if sugar intake and stress are reduced as well—they are the main contributors to breakouts.

For long-term herpes infections, it's also helpful to make dietary adjustments that increase the amount of the amino acid lysine in the diet, while reducing arginine—this disrupts the viral life cycle and makes it easier for your immune system to fight the virus. See also Immune Support and Stress.

COLD SORE COMPRESS

Makes 5 cups dried herb mix (about 50 applications)

This direct application stimulates local immunity and improves tissue quality so your body has the best chance to suppress the virus. For chicken pox or other full-body breakout, take an herb-infused bath with this same formula. Add a bit of baking soda, as it helps with the itching.

1 cup dried calendula flower
1 cup dried plantain leaf
1 cup dried chamomile flower

1 cup dried linden leaf and flower

½ cup dried self-heal leaf and flower

½ cup dried St. John's wort leaf and flower

1. In a large bowl, mix together all the herbs. Store in an airtight container.

2. Make a hot infusion: Prepare a kettle of boiling water. Measure 2 to 3 tablespoons of herbs per quart of water and place in a mason jar or French press. Pour in the boiling water, cover, and steep for 20 minutes. (Meanwhile, fill a hot water bottle.)

3. Soak a cloth in the warm tea, holding it by a dry spot and letting it cool in the air until hot but comfortable to the touch.

4. Lie down and place the wet cloth over the affected area. Cover with a dry cloth and lay the hot water bottle on top. Get comfortable and let it soak in for 10 to 20 minutes.

5. Repeat 2 to 3 times per day.

STEAM VARIATION: You can also perform a steam using these herbs as they're infusing. Simply make a blanket tent, position your face over the steaming pot, and steam yourself with these herbs for a few minutes before you sit with the compress.

COLD SORE BALM

Makes 5 ounces (about a 3-month supply)

This gentle salve is very soothing to irritated cold sores, and helps reduce inflammation while making your body's environment less hospitable to the virus.

1 fluid ounce calendula-infused oil

1 fluid ounce plantain-infused oil

½ fluid ounce self-heal–infused oil

½ fluid ounce chamomile-infused oil

½ fluid ounce St. John's wort–infused oil

½ fluid ounce thyme-infused oil

1 ounce beeswax, plus more as needed

1. Make a salve as usual (see here for complete instructions). Make it nice and soft if you'll keep it in little jars; make it slightly firmer if you're using lip balm tubes.
2. Apply liberally to the affected area 3 to 5 times daily.

High Blood Pressure/ Hypertension

Relevant tissue states: heat, tension

Relevant herbal actions: hypotensive, nervine, relaxant, sedative

Herbal Allies

- Dandelion
- Garlic
- Ginger
- Kelp
- Linden leaf and flower
- Marshmallow
- Rose
- Yarrow leaf and flower

Occasional high blood pressure is normal—it's a part of the natural response to stressful situations. Over time, though, high blood pressure can cause or worsen other cardiovascular problems. Herbs offer a nice suite of actions to reduce high blood pressure, often by addressing root causes rather than merely acting symptomatically.

It's worth noting that high blood pressure isn't always bad: New information indicates that hypertension that develops in the elder years may actually help reduce the risk of dementia. See also <u>Anxiety</u> and <u>Stress</u>.

SOFTHEARTED TEA

Makes 2 cups dried herb mix (enough for 12 to 16 quarts of tea)

Reducing stress makes a big difference, so herbs that can relax the mind while soothing the physical heart are ideal. For those with very dry constitutions, prepare this as a cold infusion instead. Drink a quart or more every day.

1 cup dried linden leaf and flower

½ cup dried marshmallow leaf

½ cup dried rose petals

1. In a small bowl, mix together all the herbs. Store in an airtight container.
2. Make a hot infusion: Prepare a kettle of boiling water. Measure 2 to 3 tablespoons of herbs per quart of water and place in a mason jar or French press. Pour in the boiling water, cover, and steep for 20 minutes or until cool enough to drink.

Hypoglycemia

Relevant tissue states: cold, damp

Relevant herbal actions: adaptogen, bitter, hepatic, insulin sensitizing

Herbal Allies

- Ashwagandha root
- Cinnamon bark
- Dandelion root
- Kelp

- Licorice root
- Milk thistle seed
- Self-heal leaf and flower
- Tulsi leaf
- St. John's wort leaf and flower

Hypoglycemia is better described as "blood sugar regulation issues," rather than simply "low blood sugar"—it is often a matter of blood sugar levels fluctuating wildly, with spikes and valleys. Ideally, we should be metabolically flexible, able to go long hours without eating and able to run smoothly while cycling through a variety of fuels. Hypoglycemia usually indicates the body is having trouble using anything except sugars and simple carbohydrates as fuel. It is closely tied to insulin resistance and diabetes and should be considered an early warning sign. The remedies here will work over time to normalize blood sugar levels and reduce hypoglycemic incidents.

Of the herbs in this book, cinnamon has the strongest activity for modulating blood sugar. As little as ½ to 2 teaspoons of cinnamon powder per day has profound effects. Combine with a couple of milk thistle capsules to boost liver function, which also improves blood sugar levels.

Reducing simple carbohydrate and sugar intake is necessary for improving blood sugar regulation. If you have sugar cravings, take a dropperful of a bitter herb tincture, like dandelion root, or sweet herb tincture, like licorice. A chromium supplement can also be helpful.

ADAPT TO BITTER
Makes 5 fluid ounces (75 to 150 doses)

This combination of adaptogens (to improve endocrine function, including blood sugar regulation) and bitters (to stimulate digestion and normalize cravings) is a good way to reset your body's internal fuel economy and help it become more flexible.

2 fluid ounces tincture of tulsi

1 fluid ounce tincture of ashwagandha

1 fluid ounce tincture of licorice

½ fluid ounce tincture of dandelion root

½ fluid ounce tincture of St. John's wort (see Tip)

1. In a small bottle, combine the tinctures. Cap the bottle and label it.

2. Take 1 to 2 droppersful 10 minutes before eating.

TIP: Omit the St. John's wort if you are concurrently taking pharmaceuticals.

STEADY STATE DECOCTION

Makes 2¾ cups dried herb mix (enough for 18 to 22 quarts of tea)

This combination provides consistent energy, keeping your body active and your mind focused without dips in vitality. Drink a quart or more over the course of the day. Effects may take some time to accumulate—stick with it.

1 cup dried ashwagandha root

½ cup dried cinnamon bark

½ cup dried dandelion root

½ cup dried kelp

¼ cup dried licorice root

1. In a small bowl, mix together all the herbs. Store in an airtight container.
2. Make a decoction: Measure 2 to 4 tablespoons of herbs per quart of water and place in a lidded pot over high heat. Add the water and cover the pot. Bring to a boil, reduce the heat, and simmer for 1 hour.
3. Strain and drink.

Hypothyroidism

Relevant tissue states: cold, dryness

Relevant herbal actions: adaptogen, carminative, nutritive, stimulant

Herbal Allies

* Angelica
* Ashwagandha root
* Ginger
* Kelp
* Licorice root
* Milk thistle seed
* St. John's wort leaf and flower
* Tulsi leaf

Hypothyroidism can be induced by hormonal imbalances (too much insulin or cortisol), by nutritional deficiencies (too little iodine), and by autoimmunity. For long-term resolution, each will need to be assessed and addressed. In the meantime, the symptoms—primarily expressions of cold and dryness—can be substantially mitigated with herbs. See also Fatigue, Hypoglycemia, and PCOS.

DEEP WARMTH ELIXIR

Makes 4 fluid ounces (60 to 120 doses)

The sweetness and warmth of this elixir will spread through the body, breaking up stagnations and building steady energy.

1 fluid ounce tincture of ashwagandha

1 fluid ounce tincture of tulsi

½ fluid ounce tincture of angelica

½ fluid ounce tincture of ginger

½ fluid ounce tincture of licorice

½ fluid ounce honey

1. In a small bottle, combine the tinctures and honey. Cap the bottle and label it.
2. Take 1 to 2 droppersful 3 to 5 times per day.

SEAWEED SNACKS

Yield varies

Roasted seaweed has a nice, crispy texture and can replace chips as a snack. The iodine content nourishes the thyroid.

Olive oil or sesame oil, for lightly coating the seaweed

2 to 3 handfuls dried kelp, cut into potato chip–size pieces (enough to make a single layer in your baking dish)

1. Preheat the oven to 350°F.
2. Spread the oil—not too much—on the kelp pieces (a mister or pastry brush is helpful here) and arrange the kelp in a single layer in a 9-by-13-inch oven-safe dish.
3. Bake for 20 minutes.
4. Store at room temperature in an airtight container and consume within 1 week.

IBS/IBD/Ulcerative Colitis

Relevant tissue states: heat (inflammation), tension

Relevant herbal actions: anti-inflammatory, astringent, demulcent, hepatic, relaxant, vulnerary

Herbal Allies

- Calendula flower
- Catnip leaf and flower
- Chamomile flower
- Fennel seed
- Ginger
- Licorice root
- Marshmallow
- Meadowsweet flower
- Peppermint leaf
- Plantain leaf
- Self-heal leaf and flower

These similar conditions have technical differences but are often conflated (both by laypersons and physicians). Fortunately, the herbal approaches we use for each are the same: soothing remedies to heal damaged tissue, relieve constriction, and calm inflammation. See also <u>Food Sensitivities</u> and <u>Leaky Gut</u>.

TESTY INTESTINES TEA

Makes 4 cups dried herb mix (enough for 24 to 32 quarts of tea)

This gently warming, relaxing blend calms the roiling and spasms that cause so much discomfort in these ailments. Drink a quart or more of tea every day.

½ cup dried catnip leaf and flower

½ cup fennel seed

½ cup dried chamomile flower

½ cup dried peppermint leaf

1/3 cup dried calendula flower

1/3 cup dried plantain leaf

1/3 cup dried tulsi leaf

¼ cup dried ginger

¼ cup dried licorice root

¼ cup dried marshmallow leaf

¼ cup dried St. John's wort leaf and flower (see Tip)

1. In a large bowl, mix together all the herbs. Store in an airtight container.

2. Make a hot infusion: Prepare a kettle of boiling water. Measure 2 to 3 tablespoons of herbs per quart of water and place in a mason jar or French press. Pour in the boiling water, cover, and steep for 20 minutes or until cool enough to drink.

TIP: Omit the St. John's wort if you are concurrently taking pharmaceuticals.

Immune Support

Relevant tissue states: cold (depressed function)

Relevant herbal actions: adaptogen, circulatory stimulant, immune stimulant, lymphatic

Herbal Allies

- Angelica
- Calendula flower
- Elder

- Elecampane root
- Garlic
- Pine
- Self-heal leaf and flower
- Thyme leaf
- Tulsi leaf

We're all exposed to lots of germs in the course of our lives, and there's little we can do about it—but we can make ourselves as resilient as possible for when we are, inevitably, exposed. Building up good host resistance or "healthy terrain" means taking care of all the body's natural defenses against infection. Deep nourishment, stress management, good sleep, and consistent movement are all critical for immune health, as this distributed system relies on the movement and refreshment of blood, lymph, and extracellular fluids to function well. See also Insomnia and Stress.

ELDER AND EVERGREEN

Makes 5 fluid ounces (75 to 150 doses)

The gentle boost to immune activity this formula provides helps stave off illness if you venture into a kindergarten classroom, airplane, or other garden of germs!

2 fluid ounces tincture of elderberry

1 fluid ounce tincture of pine

1 fluid ounce tincture of angelica or elecampane

½ fluid ounce tincture of calendula

½ fluid ounce tincture of self-heal

1. In a small bottle, combine the tinctures. Cap the bottle and label it.

2. Take 1 to 2 droppersful 3 to 5 times per day.

GARLIC ELIXIR
Makes 4 fluid ounces (30 to 60 doses)

Garlic may not seem like the most delicious of flavors, but mellowed by some honey and lifted on the aromatics of thyme and tulsi, this potent immune system stimulant gets quite a bit more palatable. This is also great as an oxymel (see here). *Note: Do not take this concurrently with pharmaceutical blood thinners.*

1 fluid ounce tincture of garlic

1 fluid ounce tincture of thyme

1 fluid ounce tincture of tulsi

1 fluid ounce garlic-infused honey

1. In a small bottle, combine the tinctures and honey. Cap the bottle and label it.
2. Take 1 to 4 droppersful 2 to 4 times per day.

Indigestion/ Dyspepsia

Relevant tissue states: cold (stagnation), tension

Relevant herbal actions: bitter, carminative, relaxant

Herbal Allies
- Catnip leaf and flower
- Chamomile flower
- Dandelion root
- Fennel seed
- Ginger
- Licorice root

- Peppermint leaf
- Sage leaf

If you're reading this book cover to cover, you've probably gathered that we like to look for the root causes of things. If you're having chronic digestive discomforts, take a hard look at your diet to see if you have any <u>food sensitivities</u>. Lucky for you, though, indigestion is a problem for which herbal quick fixes are ready at hand—read on for two simple, portable solutions.

BEFORE-MEAL BITTERS

Makes 4 fluid ounces (60 to 120 doses)

Indigestion often means just that—incomplete digestion. This formula stimulates all your digestive fluids—saliva, stomach acid, bile, and pancreatic enzymes—so digestion is as thorough and complete as possible.

1 fluid ounce tincture of dandelion root

1 fluid ounce tincture of sage

1 fluid ounce tincture of catnip

1 fluid ounce tincture of chamomile

1. In a small bottle, combine the tinctures. Cap the bottle and label it.
2. Take 1 to 2 droppersful 10 minutes before eating.

CORE CARMINATIVES

Makes 4 fluid ounces (60 to 120 doses)

This formula warms the body's core, stimulating your digestive organs and keeping the bowels from getting sluggish. If peppermint isn't your style, substitute angelica.

1½ fluid ounces tincture of ginger

1 fluid ounce tincture of fennel

1 fluid ounce tincture of peppermint (see headnote)

½ fluid ounce tincture of licorice

1. In a small bottle, combine the tinctures. Cap the bottle and label it.

2. Take 1 to 2 droppersful after each meal, or whenever your guts feel uncomfortably stuck.

Inflammation

Relevant tissue states: heat

Relevant herbal actions: adaptogen, alterative, anti-inflammatory, lymphatic

Herbal Allies

- Calendula flower
- Garlic
- Ginger
- Licorice root
- Meadowsweet flower
- Nettle leaf
- Self-heal leaf and flower
- St. John's wort leaf and flower
- Tulsi leaf
- Yarrow leaf and flower

Inflammation is an essential part of the healing process and critical to immune responses to infection. But when it is uncontrolled and goes on for too long, it can lead to serious problems: Systemic inflammation is associated with almost all chronic illnesses.

Many aspects of our modern lifestyle contribute to systemic inflammation—diets high in sugar and industrial seed oils, insufficient sleep, sedentary habits, unrelenting stress. We can transition to an "anti-inflammatory lifestyle" by making sensible, stepwise changes in these habits. And of course, in the meantime, we can work with herbs! Here we highlight some superstars well known for their capacity to reduce inflammation, no matter where in the body it occurs.

COOLING FORMULA

Makes 4½ fluid ounces (35 to 60 doses)

This combo of cooling, anti-inflammatory herbs circulates through the entire body and calms inflammation wherever it's raging.

1 fluid ounce tincture of nettle

1 fluid ounce tincture of tulsi

½ fluid ounce tincture of calendula

½ fluid ounce tincture of self-heal

⅓ fluid ounce tincture of yarrow

⅓ fluid ounce tincture of meadowsweet

⅓ fluid ounce tincture of licorice

½ fluid ounce tincture of St. John's wort (see Tip)

1. In a small bottle, combine the tinctures. Cap the bottle and label it.
2. Take 2 to 4 droppersful 3 to 5 times per day.

TIP: Omit the St. John's wort if you are concurrently taking pharmaceuticals.

COLD FIRE FORMULA

Makes 4 fluid ounces (30 to 60 doses)

Inflammation doesn't always present with surface heat signs. If you run cold but still have signs of systemic inflammation (e.g., hormonal imbalances, high cholesterol, or an elevated C-reactive protein reading on a blood test), try this formula.

1 fluid ounce tincture of ginger

1 fluid ounce tincture of garlic

½ fluid ounce tincture of tulsi

½ fluid ounce tincture of licorice

½ fluid ounce tincture of yarrow

½ fluid ounce tincture of self-heal

1. In a small bottle, combine the tinctures. Cap the bottle and label it.
2. Take 2 to 4 droppersful 3 to 5 times per day.

Insomnia

Relevant tissue states: heat (agitation), tension

Relevant herbal actions: hypnotic, relaxant, sedative

Herbal Allies

* Ashwagandha root
* Betony leaf and flower
* Catnip leaf and flower
* Chamomile flower
* Linden leaf and flower
* Rose
* Wild lettuce

Wild animals don't have insomnia. Hikers in the wilds don't either, actually. According to a 2013 study in the journal *Current Biology*, just a few days in an outdoor environment, with no

303

artificial light exposure, is enough to reestablish normal circadian rhythms—even in people who are habitual "night owls" in their city lives. This tracks with a large and growing body of evidence that indicates that our electrically lit environments are directly responsible for most sleep disturbances we experience.

Reducing evening exposure to bright lights—including TV, computer, and smartphone screens—is one of the most important steps you can take to fight insomnia. Dimming lights and avoiding screens for at least an hour before bed, and taking the herbal remedies offered here, are sure ways to improve both the quantity and quality of your sleep. See also Anxiety.

END-OF-THE-DAY ELIXIR

Makes 4 fluid ounces (60 to 120 doses)

This blend of relaxants and gentle sedatives doesn't force sleep but helps relieve the tension, anxiety, and distraction that make it difficult to transition into sleep. This formula (and any herbs taken to aid in sleep) is best taken in "pulse doses," which is much more effective than taking the total dose all at once right at bedtime. It gives the herbs time to start working in your system and emphasizes to the body that it's time to transition into sleep.

1 fluid ounce tincture of chamomile

1 fluid ounce tincture of betony

¾ fluid ounce tincture of ashwagandha

½ fluid ounce tincture of catnip

½ fluid ounce tincture of linden

¼ fluid ounce honey (plain or rose petal–infused)

1. In a small bottle, combine the tinctures and honey. Cap the bottle and label it.

2. One hour before bedtime, take 1 to 2 droppersful.
3. Thirty minutes before bedtime, take another 1 to 2 droppersful.
4. At bedtime, take the final 1 to 2 droppersful.

SLEEP!

Makes 4 fluid ounces (60 to 120 doses)

For this formula, we recruit wild lettuce, the strongest hypnotic (sleep-inducing) herb in this book. This is especially helpful if part of what's keeping you up at night is physical pain, as wild lettuce also has a pain-relieving effect. This formula, like End-of-the-Day Elixir, is best taken in "pulse doses."

2 fluid ounces tincture of wild lettuce

1 fluid ounce tincture of betony

½ fluid ounce tincture of chamomile

½ fluid ounce tincture of linden

1. In a small bottle, combine the tinctures. Cap the bottle and label it.
2. One hour before bedtime, take 1 to 2 droppersful.
3. Thirty minutes before bedtime, take another 1 to 2 droppersful.
4. At bedtime, take the final 1 to 2 droppersful.

Joint Pain

Relevant tissue states: heat (inflammation), dryness (friction), tension

Relevant herbal actions: anti-inflammatory, lubricant, relaxant, rubefacient

Herbal Allies

- Cinnamon essential oil
- Ginger
- Goldenrod leaf and flower
- Kelp
- Meadowsweet flower
- Peppermint essential oil
- Solomon's seal root

For acute or stand-alone pain in a particular joint, try one of these remedies. They'll accelerate healing if there's been an injury and reduce painful inflammation, as well.

The acronym RICE—rest, ice, compression, elevation—is a mnemonic for first aid treatments for sports injuries. The very doctor who coined this term and process, Gabe Mirkin, has actually recanted on at least the first two points. He no longer recommends either complete rest or ice applications for injuries, noting that current science shows these both delay recovery.

Gentle movement that doesn't cause pain and herbs that help increase local blood flow and speed wound healing have served us well. See also Arthritis.

JOINT LINIMENT

Makes about 8 fluid ounces (100+ applications, 30-day supply)

This liniment follows in the tradition of "hit medicine" that originated in martial arts. Warming the area, increasing blood flow, lubricating the joints, and quelling inflammation all contribute to the overall effect.

Healing joint pain is best done with both inside-out and outside-in remedies. For the internal side of things, check out Joint Support Decoction.

4 fluid ounces ginger-infused oil

2 fluid ounces Solomon's seal–infused oil, or tincture of Solomon's seal

2 fluid ounces tincture of meadowsweet

80 drops peppermint essential oil or cinnamon essential oil (or both!)

1. In a small bottle, combine the infused oils, tincture, and essential oil(s). Cap the bottle and label it, including *Shake well before each use*.
2. Hold your palm over the bottle's mouth and tilt it to deposit a small amount in your palm. Rub between your hands to warm the treatment, and apply to the painful joints.
3. Massage the liniment into the joints until your hands no longer feel oily. Really work the liniment into the tissue—rubbing helps in its own right.
4. Repeat the application 3 to 5 times per day. More is better!

KELP WRAP

Makes 1 application

Seaweed is very mineral rich, and, surprisingly, much of this nutrient content can be absorbed directly through the skin to accelerate wound healing at an injury site. Kelp also serves to reduce pain and inflammation when applied this way.

1 strip dried kelp (long enough to cover the injured area)

Hot water bottle, for warming (optional)

1. Drop the kelp into a pot of hot (not boiling) water. It will rehydrate and become soft and pliable.
2. Remove it from the water and wrap the still-warm kelp around the joint that hurts.

3. Cover with a cloth or towel and hold a hot water bottle against it, if desired. Leave in place for 20 minutes.

4. Repeat 2 to 3 times per day for best effects.

POULTICE VARIATION: If your kelp is already chopped, make a poultice instead—a warm, wet mass of rehydrated kelp—and apply to the affected area.

Leaky Gut

Relevant tissue states: laxity (barrier compromise), heat (inflammation)
Relevant herbal actions: astringent, vulnerary

Herbal Allies

- Calendula flower
- Goldenrod leaf and flower
- Marshmallow
- Meadowsweet flower
- Plantain leaf
- Self-heal leaf and flower
- Yarrow leaf and flower

Leaky gut syndrome is often due to dysbiosis, because unfriendly microorganisms in the intestines secrete toxins that damage the intestinal lining's cells. Leaky gut is also a common result of food sensitivities, as the inflammatory response to the allergenic food weakens the lining of the intestines. At the same time, it's a major contributor to food sensitivities, because compromised barriers allow various undigested food proteins through; the immune system regards these as potentially dangerous and mounts an inflammatory response—and now this food is a new trigger. As you might imagine, this vicious cycle often leads to an ever-dwindling set of "safe" foods.

Correcting leaky gut is a critical aspect of long-term digestive (and whole-body) health. See also Food Sensitivities and IBS/IBD/Ulcerative Colitis.

Good vitamin D status is essential for many aspects of health, including gut integrity. Vitamin D helps keep the "tight junctions" in the intestinal wall at a proper degree of permeability—not too loose, not too tight. For most Americans, a daily vitamin D dose of 5,000 IU is necessary to maintain adequate levels.

BARRIER INTEGRI-TEA

Makes 4 cups dried herb mix (enough for 21 to 32 quarts of tea)

These gentle, tissue-tightening, wound-healing herbs help the intestinal mucous membranes achieve a healthy degree of integrity once again. Drink a quart or more every day.

1 cup dried calendula flower

1 cup dried plantain leaf

½ cup dried goldenrod leaf and flower

½ cup dried meadowsweet flower

½ cup dried self-heal leaf and flower

½ cup dried yarrow leaf and flower

1. In a medium bowl, mix together all the herbs. Store in an airtight container.
2. Make a hot infusion: Prepare a kettle of boiling water. Measure 2 to 3 tablespoons of herbs per quart of water and place in a mason jar or French press. Pour in the boiling water, cover, and steep for 20 minutes or until cool enough to drink.

HONEY PASTE

Makes about 1 cup (18 to 40 doses)

An herbal powder honey paste is a good delivery method to target the intestines—the powdered herbs travel deep in the GI tract before being absorbed. You can stir this into tea or hot cereal, or just eat it off the spoon!

¾ cup honey

4 teaspoons powdered marshmallow root

1 teaspoon powdered calendula flower

1 teaspoon powdered plantain leaf

1 teaspoon powdered goldenrod leaf and flower

1 teaspoon powdered self-heal leaf and flower

1. Put the honey in a jar and warm it gently by placing the jar in a small pot of hot (not boiling) water on the stove or on a hot plate. (Don't let water get into the jar; keep the water level in the pot 1 to 2 inches below the mouth of the jar.) As the honey warms, a moment will occur when it transitions suddenly to a thin, watery consistency. When this happens, turn off the heat and stir the powdered herbs into the honey.

2. Stir very, very well, even for a few extra minutes after you think it's all stirred in, so it will not separate or clump as it cools. The paste will thicken as it cools and even more over time.

3. Take 1 to 3 teaspoons 3 times per day.

Menopause/ Andropause

Relevant tissue states: cold (stagnation)

Relevant herbal actions: adaptogen, alterative, cholagogue, hepatic, nutritive

Herbal Allies

- Ashwagandha root
- Calendula flower
- Kelp
- Licorice root
- Milk thistle seed
- Nettle leaf
- Sage leaf
- Self-heal leaf and flower
- St. John's wort leaf and flower
- Tulsi leaf

During menopause and andropause, the gonads (ovaries, testes) begin to decline in activity. Meanwhile, the adrenal glands take on the responsibility of producing estrogen, progesterone, testosterone, and other hormones. When this process is unruly or uncomfortable, it generally boils down to either liver deficiency or overload, or adrenal depletion.

Many people looking for phytoestrogens try soy, clover, or hops supplements. Those looking for phytoandrogens often try pine pollen extracts or any of a thousand other "natural testosterone solutions." But these don't work the same way pharmaceutical hormone replacements do. In either case, if your fundamentals aren't lined up, it'll be slow going. First, build good self-care habits around food, sleep, stress, and movement; then address major confounding issues such as impaired detoxification (see here), Hypoglycemia, Inflammation, and Stress; and then see what remains.

SAGE AND WISDOM FORMULA
Makes 2 fluid ounces (30 to 60 doses)

Sage is famed for its ability to calm night sweats, a common issue in the transition to elderhood. (This is likely as much to do with its stimulating effects on liver function as with any phytoestrogenic activity.) Combining sage with adaptogens deepens the effect on hormonal balance.

1 fluid ounce tincture of sage

⅓ fluid ounce tincture of ashwagandha

⅓ fluid ounce tincture of licorice

⅓ fluid ounce tincture of tulsi

1. In a small bottle, combine the tinctures. Cap the bottle and label it.
2. Take 1 to 2 droppersful 3 to 5 times per day.

HEPATICLEAR

Makes 2½ cups dried herb mix (enough for 14 to 20 quarts of tea)

This tea blend gets the liver going and clears out stagnant fluids in the body—supporting good blood "filtration" to eliminate excessive hormones. Drink a quart or more every day.

1 cup dried calendula flower

½ cup dried tulsi leaf

½ cup dried self-heal leaf and flower

¼ cup dried licorice root

¼ cup St. John's wort leaf and flower (see Tip)

1. In a small bowl, mix together all the herbs. Store in an airtight container.
2. Make a hot infusion: Prepare a kettle of boiling water. Measure 2 to 3 tablespoons of herbs per quart of water and

place in a mason jar or French press. Pour in the boiling water, cover, and steep for 20 minutes or until cool enough to drink.

TIP: Omit the St. John's wort if you are concurrently taking pharmaceuticals.

Menstrual Cycle Irregularities

Relevant tissue states: cold (stagnation), laxity

Relevant herbal actions: astringent, carminative, circulatory stimulant, emmenagogue, nutritive, rubefacient

Herbal Allies

* Angelica
* Ashwagandha root
* Betony leaf and flower
* Chamomile flower
* Dandelion leaf
* Ginger
* Goldenrod leaf and flower
* Kelp
* Milk thistle seed
* Nettle leaf
* Sage leaf
* Self-heal leaf and flower
* Tulsi leaf

This includes various disruptions of the menstrual cycle. Each is addressed slightly differently, but a few overarching actions emerge that help with all of them: nourishing the body, improving circulation, and stimulating the liver and kidneys to clear away used-up hormones.

Delayed or absent menses may be due to a lack of adequate nourishment, especially protein, or to disruptions in hormone levels. (Sometimes these share a cause. A high-sugar diet is nutrient-poor, and the havoc it wreaks on blood sugar levels has a cascade effect that disrupts hormone balance. Stress makes us tend to eat gratifying but poor-quality food, and excessive stress-response hormones interfere with the normal actions of estrogen and progesterone.)

Irregular cycles, with no predictable pattern, may also be due to poor nourishment, liver stagnation or strain, or an irregular lifestyle—especially erratic sleep habits. The daily cycle shapes the monthly cycle, like small and large gears interlocking in a watch.

Overheavy bleeding generally comes from hormones not clearing efficiently at the liver, though it may also be connected with the development of fibroids or polyps. If heavy bleeding persists, seek medical attention.

See also PCOS, Endometriosis, and PMS.

STEADY CYCLE TEA

Makes 3½ cups dried herb mix (enough for 20 to 28 quarts of tea)

These herbs provide substantial nourishment and a bit of gentle kidney, lymphatic, and endocrine stimulation. Long-term use of a formula like this has been the major factor in improvement for a great many of our clients with menstrual irregularities of all types. Add ginger if you run cold, betony if you're frequently anxious, and peppermint for taste (if you like it). Drink a quart or more every day.

1 cup dried nettle leaf
1 cup dried dandelion leaf

½ cup dried goldenrod leaf and flower

½ cup dried self-heal leaf and flower

¼ cup dried tulsi leaf

¼ cup dried kelp

1. In a small bowl, mix together all the herbs. Store in an airtight container.
2. Make a long infusion: Prepare a kettle of boiling water. Measure 2 to 3 tablespoons of herbs per quart of water and place in a mason jar or French press. Pour in the boiling water, cover, and steep for 8 hours or overnight.

BLEEDY TEA

Makes 3 cups dried herb mix (enough for 20 to 26 quarts of tea)

To bring on menstruation, drink this tea for 3 days to 1 week prior to the expected start of your next period. Drink this tea very hot for best results. Reheat as necessary, and drink a quart or more over the course of the day. For a stronger effect, take a dropperful of angelica tincture together with each cup of tea.

1 cup dried chamomile flower

1 cup dried tulsi leaf

⅓ cup dried goldenrod leaf and flower

⅓ cup dried ginger

⅓ cup dried angelica root

1. In a small bowl, mix together all the herbs. Store in an airtight container.
2. Make a hot infusion: Prepare a kettle of boiling water. Measure 2 to 3 tablespoons of herbs per quart of water and place in a mason jar or French press. Pour in the boiling water, cover, and steep for 20 minutes or until cool enough to drink.

Muscle Soreness/ Post-Workout Recovery

Relevant tissue states: heat (inflammation), tension

Relevant herbal actions: anodyne, nervous trophorestorative, relaxant, rubefacient

Herbal Allies

- Cinnamon bark
- Ginger
- Goldenrod leaf and flower
- Meadowsweet flower
- Peppermint essential oil
- Wild lettuce
- Yarrow leaf and flower

A bit of delayed-onset muscle soreness after a hard day's work or an intense workout is normal. Rest well! Recovery time is when muscles grow stronger; if you don't give them time to recover fully, you'll confound your efforts. Eat well, too— providing the necessary nutrients speeds recovery. Bone broth with seaweed added is a great place to start (see Build-Up Broth).

MUSCLE RUB

Makes 8 fluid ounces (100+ applications, 30-day supply)

These warming herbs increase local circulation, simultaneously reducing inflammation and soothing tension. If, after applications, you're still in a lot of pain when it's time to go to bed, take 1 to 2 droppersful of wild lettuce tincture for further relief.

2 fluid ounces ginger-infused oil

2 fluid ounces goldenrod-infused oil

2 fluid ounces tincture of ginger

2 fluid ounces tincture of meadowsweet

80 drops peppermint essential oil or cinnamon essential oil (or both!)

1. In a small bottle, combine the infused oils, tinctures, and essential oil(s). Cap the bottle and label it, including *Shake well before each use*.
2. Hold your palm over the bottle's mouth and tilt to deposit a small amount in your palm. Rub between your hands to warm the treatment, and apply to the painful joints.
3. Massage the liniment into the joints until your hands no longer feel oily. Really work the liniment into the tissue.
4. Repeat the application 3 to 5 times per day. More is better!

Nausea

Relevant tissue states: heat (agitation), tension (spasm)

Relevant herbal actions: antiemetic, carminative, relaxant

Herbal Allies

- Catnip leaf and flower
- Chamomile flower
- Fennel seed
- Ginger
- Peppermint leaf

One way or another, nausea almost always comes from food—a sensitivity, some indigestion, various potential infections. Especially if nausea happens frequently, look closely at your diet—keeping a journal can be helpful—to identify any patterns that occur around its appearance. Maybe when you eat on the run, or eat wheat products, or have really fiery spices —whatever it is for you, the only way to identify it is to pay attention in an organized way.

After a bout of vomiting, some warm, slightly weak Calm Core Tea can be the easiest thing to drink for quite some time. Then slowly reintroduce broth, then soup, then stew … gradually progressing from food prepared to be very warm andmoist to food that is more cool and dry, like salad.

Both of the following formulas are also excellent for morning sickness. If you feel you can't get anything down at all, just one drop of ginger tincture all by itself on the tongue can be helpful, or even just smelling strong ginger tea.

CALM CORE TEA

Makes 3¼ cups dried herb mix (enough for 20 to 26 quarts of tea)

For most cases of nausea, this combination of the best herbal antiemetics should help very quickly. If you know you prefer (or dislike) the flavor of one of these ingredients, feel free to adjust its proportion. This also helps as a preventive—if prone to nausea, drink a quart or more every day.

1 cup dried catnip leaf and flower
1 cup dried chamomile flower
½ cup dried peppermint leaf
½ cup fennel seed
¼ cup dried ginger

1. In a medium bowl, mix together all the herbs. Store in an airtight container.

2. Make a hot infusion: Prepare a kettle of boiling water. Measure 2 to 3 tablespoons of herbs per quart of water and place in a mason jar or French press. Pour in the boiling water, cover, and steep for 20 minutes or until cool enough to drink.

3. Drink a cupful, slowly, in small sips. If the nausea is very severe, just sit for a while and inhale the scent rising off the hot tea.

GENTLE GINGER ELIXIR

Makes 5 fluid ounces (60 to 120 doses)

This elixir is one to keep in your herbal first aid kit at all times. You never know when nausea will strike, and a quick herbal relief will be very welcome. Make this with ginger-infused honey if you have the time to prepare that in advance.

2 fluid ounces tincture of ginger

1 fluid ounce tincture of catnip

1 fluid ounce tincture of chamomile

1 fluid ounce honey

1. In a small bottle, combine all the ingredients. Cap the bottle and label it.

2. Take 1 to 2 droppersful every 20 minutes until relief occurs.

Pain Management

Relevant tissue states: varies substantially with each presentation
Relevant herbal actions: analgesic, anodyne, anti-inflammatory, circulatory stimulant, lymphatic, relaxant

Herbal Allies

- Chamomile flower
- Ginger

- Kelp
- Meadowsweet flower
- Tulsi leaf
- Wild lettuce

Pain is not one thing; pain is complex. This is true even at a high level of abstraction. Things known to increase systemic inflammation and exacerbate pain wherever it occurs in the body include food sensitivities, depression, sedentation, insomnia, stress—each a nearly universal burden on our population. Pain is also complex in each instance, variously composed of inflammation, swelling, constriction, pressure, and spasms.

Anytime this many causes and factors influence a situation, we might be inclined toward frustration or despair—"It's too big to fix!" But this also means we have many avenues of approach to try resolving the problem. Aside from rational lifestyle changes to move more, sleep better, and so on, it's also known that meditation, acupuncture, and even simple warmth can increase endorphins—our internal painkillers. Gentle touch can "distract" the nerves carrying the pain signal to the brain, reducing its intensity. And herbs can address each of the disordered tissue states contributing to the pain.

When pain is chronic, it is essential to sort out the hot vs. cold, dry vs. damp, and tense vs. lax aspects of the presentation and adjust herbal formulas accordingly.

DAYTIME PAIN COMBO
Makes 7 fluid ounces (50 to 90 doses)

Take this tincture blend consistently for best effects; you'll feel different by the time you need to refill, but only if you stick to your dosing schedule. You need the signals these herbs give the body to reach a saturation point and sustain it.

4 fluid ounces tincture of tulsi

2 fluid ounces tincture of meadowsweet

1 fluid ounce tincture of ginger

1. In a small bottle, combine the tinctures. Cap the bottle and label it.
2. Take 2 to 4 droppersful 3 to 5 times per day.

NIGHTTIME PAIN COMBO

Makes 7 fluid ounces (100 to 150 doses)

Wild lettuce is here for you. Switch to this formula an hour or two before bed so its effects can soak in and peak as you transition into sleep. Keep it near the bed in case you wake up during the night. This formula (and any herbs taken to aid sleep) is best taken in "pulse doses," which are more effective than taking the full dose at once right at bedtime. This gives the herbs time to start working in your system and reminds your body it's time to transition into sleep.

3 fluid ounces tincture of wild lettuce

2 fluid ounces tincture of chamomile

1 fluid ounce tincture of ginger

1 fluid ounce tincture of meadowsweet

1. In a small bottle, combine the tinctures. Cap the bottle and label it.
2. One hour before bedtime, take 1 to 2 droppersful.
3. Thirty minutes before bedtime, take another 1 to 2 droppersful.
4. At bedtime, take the final 1 to 2 droppersful.

PCOS

Relevant tissue states: cold (stagnation), dampness
Relevant herbal actions: adaptogen, alterative, cholagogue, diuretic, hepatic, hypoglycemic lymphatic, nutritive

Herbal Allies

- Cinnamon bark
- Dandelion leaf
- Goldenrod leaf and flower
- Milk thistle seed
- Nettle leaf
- Self-heal leaf and flower
- St. John's wort leaf and flower
- Tulsi leaf

PCOS stands for "polycystic ovarian syndrome," although not everyone diagnosed with PCOS actually has cysts. Its symptoms might include irregular menstrual cycles, excessively high levels of sex hormones (including both estrogen and testosterone), facial and body hair growth, and infertility. Ovaries are extremely sensitive to fluctuations in insulin, a hormone that regulates blood sugar, and there is a strong correlation between PCOS and uncontrolled blood sugar levels. When insulin levels are high and the system becomes overworked while coping with that, other hormones may become elevated in the body.

REGULATE AND ELIMINATE

Makes 3½ cups dried herb mix (enough for 20 to 28 quarts of tea)

This tea has two goals: improve the regulation of blood sugar and accelerate the elimination of hormonal "trash." Drink a quart or more every day.

1 cup dried tulsi leaf

1 cup dried self-heal leaf and flower

1/3 cup dried dandelion leaf

1/3 cup dried nettle leaf

1/3 cup dried goldenrod leaf and flower

¼ cup dried cinnamon bark

¼ cup dried St. John's wort leaf and flower (see Tip)

1. In a medium bowl, mix together all the herbs. Store in an airtight container.
2. Make a long infusion: Prepare a kettle of boiling water. Measure 2 to 3 tablespoons of herbs per quart of water and place in a mason jar or French press. Pour in the boiling water, cover, and steep for 8 hours or overnight.

TIP: Omit the St. John's wort if you are concurrently taking pharmaceuticals.

MAINTENANCE MORSELS

Makes about 24 pieces

With a decent amount of protein and low amounts of carbohydrates, these make a great snack to help you avoid eating sugary things between meals. This is a key way to improve blood sugar regulation; plus, these herbs help with insulin sensitivity and hormonal balance, too!

1/3 cup powdered cinnamon

1/3 cup powdered milk thistle

1/3 cup powdered nettle leaf

3 tablespoons powdered tulsi leaf or St. John's wort leaf and
flower (see Tip)

¾ cup nut butter

½ cup honey

Unsweetened shredded coconut, cocoa powder, powdered
cinnamon, ginger, cayenne, or whatever seems tasty to you,
for coating

1. In a medium bowl, blend the powders together.
2. Add the nut butter and honey. Stir to combine and form a
   thick "dough."
3. Roll the dough into 1-inch balls, then roll in your coating of
   choice.
4. Eat 1 to 4 per day.

TIP: Do not use the St. John's wort if you are concurrently
taking pharmaceuticals.

PMS

Relevant tissue states: cold, dampness (stagnation), tension
Relevant herbal actions: adaptogen, antispasmodic, diuretic,
hepatic, nervine

Herbal Allies

- Angelica
- Ashwagandha root
- Betony leaf and flower
- Chamomile flower
- Dandelion
- Elderflower
- Ginger
- Goldenrod leaf and flower

- Linden leaf and flower
- Milk thistle seed
- Sage leaf
- Self-heal leaf and flower
- Rose
- St. John's wort leaf and flower
- Tulsi leaf
- Yarrow leaf and flower

PMS can have both emotional and physical symptoms. These tend to overlap when viewed as patterns—*coldness* can present as both mental depression and the physical stagnation of sluggish menses, for instance. This means that addressing the physical often takes care of the emotional, and vice versa.

Because PMS can manifest in different ways for different people, many herbs have the potential to help. Experiment to find your favorites, but start with herbs that warm the core, increase flow, and support eliminatory organs such as the liver and kidneys.

During menarche (when menses first begin in adolescence), it's normal for the period to be a little unpredictable and for pains to occur. These formulas help normalize the cycle and reduce PMS symptoms. See also Menstrual Cycle Irregularities.

GLOW WITH THE FLOW TEA

Makes 3¾ cups dried herb mix (enough for 24 to 30 quarts of tea)

For cramping, bloating, kidney pain, and exhaustion, as well as frustration, depression, and irritability, this tea is a winner. Drink this tea every day in the week before menstruation, and continue during menstruation, if desired. (In fact, you could just drink it every day of the month—it's that tasty!) For a deeper effect, take a dropperful of ashwagandha tincture and a capsule of powdered milk thistle with each cup of tea.

1 cup dried tulsi leaf

½ cup dried betony leaf and flower

½ cup dried chamomile flower

½ cup dried elderflower

½ cup dried linden leaf and flower

¼ cup dried ginger

¼ cup dried rose petals

¼ cup dried St. John's wort leaf and flower (see Tip)

1. In a medium bowl, mix together all the herbs. Store in an airtight container.
2. Make a hot infusion: Prepare a kettle of boiling water. Measure 2 to 3 tablespoons of herbs per quart of water and place in a mason jar or French press. Pour in the boiling water, cover, and steep for 20 minutes or longer.
3. Drink a quart or more over the course of the day.

TIP: Omit the St. John's wort if you are concurrently taking pharmaceuticals.

PMS ELIXIR

Makes 3¾ fluid ounces (50 to 80 doses)

This helps stir up the pelvic blood and lymph, warm the core and release constrictions there, and settle difficult emotions.

1 fluid ounce tincture of chamomile

1 fluid ounce tincture of self-heal

⅓ fluid ounce tincture of dandelion

⅓ fluid ounce tincture of goldenrod

⅓ fluid ounce tincture of sage

¼ fluid ounce tincture of angelica (see Tip)

¼ fluid ounce tincture of ginger

¼ fluid ounce honey

1. In a small bottle, combine the tinctures and the honey. Cap the bottle and label it.

2. Take 1 to 2 droppersful 3 to 5 times per day.

TIP: If you typically have very heavy flow, omit the angelica and reduce the ginger by half.

Postpartum Support

Relevant tissue states: cold (depletion, stagnation)

Relevant herbal actions: adaptogen, alterative, hepatic, nutritive

Herbal Allies

- Dandelion root
- Kelp
- Milk thistle seed
- Nettle leaf
- St. John's wort leaf and flower
- Tulsi leaf

Growing a baby and giving birth is an exhausting and depleting process, and for many mothers, it's immediately followed by another depleting and exhausting process—lactation. The process of labor and delivery also includes intense hormonal changes, which absolutely have emotional as well as physical effects. Traditional postpartum support efforts focused on deep nutrition and herbs for liver support as a foundation for recovery, and ours do, too!

BACK TO BASELINE TEA

Makes 2 cups dried herb mix (enough for 12 to 16 quarts of tea)

Especially for someone who had trouble conceiving, who is insulin-resistant, or who has other hormonal issues, the liver is the first place to focus. You can't get back to baseline, mentally or hormonally, until the liver is able to restore normal levels.

St. John's wort stimulates the liver and speeds clearance of hormones ready to be broken down. It also increases production and uptake of neurotransmitters such as serotonin in the enteric nervous system. Between this and its slight bitterness, St. John's wort improves digestive function—often a site of sluggishness for pregnant people and new mothers.

If St. John's wort is contraindicated (i.e., if mom or baby take prescription medications), work with powdered milk thistle capsules or dandelion root tincture, along with tulsi infusions, instead. Feel free to add any flavor herbs, either to the mixture or on a cup-by-cup basis. Peppermint, fennel, chamomile, pine, sage, and ginger are all compatible flavors. Drink a quart or more every day.

1 cup dried St. John's wort leaf and flower
1 cup dried tulsi leaf

1. In a small bowl, mix together the herbs. Store in an airtight container.
2. Make a hot infusion: Prepare a kettle of boiling water. Measure 2 to 3 tablespoons of herbs per quart of water and place in a mason jar or French press. Pour in the boiling water, cover, and steep for 20 minutes or until cool enough to drink.

NUTRITIVE AND ADAPTOGENIC REMEDIES

See the recipes for <u>Nettle and Friends Tea</u>, <u>Build-Up Broth</u>, <u>Add Apt Aid</u>, and <u>Morale Morsels</u>. Each can be extremely helpful for rebuilding nutrient stores after giving birth or while breastfeeding.

Rash

Relevant tissue states: heat (inflammation), dryness or dampness, laxity

Relevant herbal actions: anti-inflammatory, astringent, demulcent

Herbal Allies

* Calendula flower
* Kelp
* Licorice root
* Plantain leaf
* Rose
* Self-heal leaf and flower
* St. John's wort leaf and flower
* Uva-ursi leaf
* Yarrow leaf and flower

A sudden appearance of a rash generally means you've come into contact with some kind of irritant—an irritating plant, a toxic chemical, or perhaps an insect bite or sting. Wash the area well with soap and water. Then apply insights from basic herbal energetics: If the rash is dry, use moistening herbs and preparations; if it's damp and oozy, use drying agents.

   If there doesn't seem to have been any contact with an irritating plant, chemical, or other direct trigger, the rash may be an external reflection of an internal imbalance. Allergies can cause this, of course, as well as overworked internal detoxification systems. See Allergies, Bites and Stings, and Detox.

DRY RASH SALVE
Makes 9 ounces (60-day supply)

Salves are emollient due to their oil and wax content, especially when they have a moisturizing oil, like olive oil, as the base. In this simple formula, the herbs' healing and anti-inflammatory effects enhance the emollient effect.

3 fluid ounces calendula-infused oil

3 fluid ounces plantain-infused oil

2 fluid ounces licorice-infused oil

1 ounce beeswax, plus more as needed

1. Prepare a salve as usual (see here for complete instructions).
2. Gently apply a thin layer to the affected area at least twice a day.

WEEPY RASH POULTICE
Makes 4½ cups dried herb mix (enough for 12 to 18 poultices)

Contact with poison ivy and similar plants often produces a rash with fluid-filled blisters. These call for astringents, and those are best delivered in a water extract—a poultice or compress.

Learn to identify the plants that cause contact rash in your area! Poison ivy, poison oak, and poison sumac all grow in the US. Check out poison-ivy.org for great pictures and details about how to make a positive identification, as well as how to tell them apart from benign look-alike plants.

1 cup dried calendula flower

1 cup dried rose petals

1 cup dried self-heal leaf and flower

½ cup dried St. John's wort leaf and flower

½ cup dried uva-ursi leaf

½ cup dried yarrow leaf and flower

Boiling water, to make the poultice

1. In a large bowl, mix together all the herbs. Store in an airtight container.
2. Measure 4 to 6 tablespoons of the herb mixture and place in a heat-proof dish.
3. Pour just enough boiling water over the herbs to get them fully saturated—not so much that they're swimming. Let the herbs soak for 5 minutes.
4. Apply the mass of herbs, warm and wet, to the affected area. Cover with a cloth. Keep in place for 5 to 10 minutes, then gently pat dry.
5. Repeat 1 to 3 times per day.

TIP: If you don't have these herbs on hand, plain green or black tea bags will do the trick! Just get them warm and wet, apply them over the rash, and let them sit in place for 20 minutes.

Seasonal Depression

Relevant tissue states: cold (depression)

Relevant herbal actions: exhilarant, nervine, stimulant

Herbal Allies

- Angelica
- Ashwagandha root
- Calendula flower

- Dandelion flower
- Ginger
- Goldenrod leaf and flower
- St. John's wort leaf and flower
- Tulsi leaf

When the sun is low and the skies are grey, most everyone feels a little less enthusiastic about customer service and commuting. There's no mystery here! When these feelings become obtrusive, we call it depression. But what if that's not quite it? Ancestrally, it's completely normal for us to have "hibernatory" behavior in winter, as the light wanes. Vitamin D levels decline, too, which affects multiple hormonal patterns in the body. When these internal, seasonal shifts run up against external social norms—the expectation that we should all be homogenous in output, attitude, and behavior throughout the various seasons —it can be easy for something normal to become pathologized.

Does that mean nothing is wrong? Well, if you're hibernating and feel good about it, nothing's wrong! But if you're hibernating and feel despondent about it, you should fine-tune things, both in your body and outlook. Herbs are an ideal ally for this. See also Depression.

SOLSTICE ELIXIR

Makes 8 fluid ounces (many doses)

This is a bottle of sunshine. Plan ahead! Make this at summer solstice with fresh plant matter for optimal results. If you have the chance, infuse your honey with freshly gathered linden flowers for 1 month before making this formula. It's divine!

4 fluid ounces tincture of dandelion flower

1½ fluid ounces tincture of calendula

1½ fluid ounces tincture of tulsi

½ fluid ounce tincture of St. John's wort (see Tip)

½ fluid ounce honey

1. In a small bottle, combine the tinctures and honey. Cap the bottle and label it.
2. Take 1 to 2 droppersful 3 to 5 times per day, plus more as needed.

TIP: Omit the St. John's wort if you are concurrently taking pharmaceuticals.

SUNNY TEA

Makes 2½ cups dried herb mix (enough for 14 to 20 quarts of tea)

Warming, uplifting, and exhilarating, this formula wakes up your brain and helps you remember the sunlight, even when clouds are in the way. Feel free to add ½ cup of your favorite aromatic herbs—catnip, chamomile, peppermint, even sage or thyme— whatever tastes good to you! We want this tea to be a source of delight. Drink a quart or more every day.

1 cup dried tulsi leaf

½ cup dried calendula flower

½ cup dried goldenrod leaf and flower

¼ cup dried ginger

¼ cup dried St. John's wort leaf and flower (see Tip)

1. In a small bowl, mix together all the herbs. Store in an airtight container.
2. Make a hot infusion: Prepare a kettle of boiling water. Measure 2 to 3 tablespoons of herbs per quart of water and

place in a mason jar or French press. Pour in the boiling water, cover, and steep for 20 minutes or until cool enough to drink.

TIP: Omit the St. John's wort if you are concurrently taking pharmaceuticals.

Sinusitis/Stuffy Nose

Relevant tissue states: heat (inflammation), laxity (mucous membranes)

Relevant herbal actions: antifungal, anti-inflammatory, antimicrobial, astringent, decongestant, demulcent

Herbal Allies

- Calendula flower
- Garlic
- Goldenrod leaf and flower
- Pine
- Marshmallow
- Sage leaf
- Thyme leaf
- Uva-ursi leaf

Runny nose is a vital response to a cold or the flu! Believe it or not, mucus is actually full of antibodies. Drying it up with pharmaceutical decongestants makes the tissue more susceptible to infection. Keeping mucous membranes at a happy medium—not too dry, not too drippy—helps shorten the illness and prevent complications.

If not connected to a full respiratory infection, or if chronic or recurrent, the cause of symptoms is likely a complex of bacterial, fungal, and viral components. (This is why it can persist even after multiple rounds of antibiotics.) Antimicrobial herbs are less specific than antibiotic drugs, which is a benefit in this

334

case, meaning that they can counteract a variety of pathogens and compromised states simultaneously.

Grating fresh horseradish and breathing its fumes, or eating prepared horseradish or wasabi, is a great way to clear the sinuses. If you've been blowing your nose a lot and the skin is irritated, some soft, simple salve or lanolin is very soothing.

See also Fire Cider, Cold and Flu, and Immune Support.

SINUS-CLEARING STEAM

Makes 2 cups dried herb mix (enough for 4 to 8 steams)

Steaming is a universal treatment across cultures for any respiratory system troubles, including those related to the sinuses. The combination of hot steam and the evaporating volatile oils from the herbs makes it very difficult for pathogens to survive and stimulates immune response in the mucous membranes.

1 cup dried pine needles

½ cup dried sage leaf

½ cup dried thyme leaf

½ gallon water

5 garlic cloves, chopped, per steam (optional)

1. In a small bowl, mix the pine, sage, and thyme. Store in an airtight container.

2. Make and execute an herbal steam: In a medium pot over high heat, boil the water. Place the pot on a heat-proof surface, someplace where you can sit near it, and make a tent with a blanket or towel. Add ¼ to ½ cup of the herb mixture to the water, along with the garlic (if using). Position your face over the steam and remain there for 5 to 20 minutes. (Bring a handkerchief, your nose will run as your sinuses clear!)

3. Repeat 2 to 3 times per day.

TIP: Similar microbe-clearing benefits can be gained by working with aromatic herbs as incense or a smudge stick (a tightly wrapped bundle of leaves, lit on one end to produce medicinal smoke). A study by Nautiyal et al. in the *Journal of Ethnopharmacology* found that "[when] using medicinal smoke[,] it is possible to completely eliminate diverse plant and human pathogenic bacteria of the air within confined space." Conifer trees like pine are particularly good at this.

Sore Throat

Relevant tissue states: heat (inflammation), dryness or dampness
Relevant herbal actions: anti-inflammatory, antimicrobial, astringent, demulcent, mucous membrane tonic

Herbal Allies

- Cinnamon bark
- Ginger
- Goldenrod leaf and flower
- Licorice root
- Marshmallow
- Sage leaf
- Self-heal leaf and flower

Sore throats are generally due to infection, whether that's a simple cold, the flu, or strep throat. When choosing remedies, it is helpful to differentiate between the hot, inflamed, *dry* sore throat and the cold, *wet* sore throat induced by post-nasal drip. Use extra demulcents for the former and astringent mucous membrane tonics for the latter. See also Cold and Flu and Immune Support.

SORE THROAT TEA

Makes 2 cups dried herb mix (enough for 12 to 16 quarts of tea)

We make this perennial favorite in a big batch every winter. Ryn's particularly prone to sore throat—it's his early warning sign of a cold coming on—and if he starts with this tea right away, it can cut the sickness short before it gets going.

Add any spices you like, such as allspice, clove, or star anise. You can also include orange peel—simply chop the peel of your (organic!) oranges, and let dry fully before adding.

Stir in some lemon and honey if you like the flavors. Lemon has some antimicrobial action, and the sour and sweet flavors both stimulate the flow of healthy mucus, which fights infection. You can also add a bit of butter, ghee, or coconut oil—just a ½ teaspoon or so per cup of hot tea. The medium-chain fatty acids (MCFAs) in these oils are topically antimicrobial, and add a nice "coating" quality to the drink.

1 cup marshmallow root

½ cup dried ginger

¼ cup dried cinnamon bark

¼ cup dried licorice root

1. In a small bowl, mix together all the herbs. Store in an airtight container.

2. Make a decoction: Measure 2 to 4 tablespoons of herbs per quart of water and place in a lidded pot over high heat. Add the water and cover the pot. Bring to a boil, reduce the heat, and simmer for 1 hour.

3. To enhance the soothing effects of the mucilaginous herbs in this blend, cool the tea fully after decoction, then continue to

cool for 1 to 2 more hours. Strain, and reheat before drinking.

4. Drink liberally throughout the day.

HERB GARGLE

Makes 16 fluid ounces (enough for several gargles)

Sage is an aromatic astringent, and it specifically kills rhinovirus —a virus that causes many colds. Combining it with vinegar and salt enhances these properties. If you have a dry sore throat, you may want to follow this with a nice cup of marshmallow tea.

8 fluid ounces water

2 tablespoons dried sage leaf

8 fluid ounces apple cider vinegar

3 teaspoons salt

1. In a small pot over high heat, bring the water to a boil. Remove it from the heat and add the sage. Cover tightly and let infuse for 20 minutes.

2. Strain the liquid into a pint-size mason jar.

3. Add the vinegar and salt, cover the jar, and shake well.

4. Pour off 1 fluid ounce or so and gargle with it for 2 to 3 minutes. Rinse your mouth out with water afterward—the vinegar's acidity can wear down tooth enamel if left in place.

5. Repeat 3 to 5 times per day.

Sprains and Strains

Relevant tissue states: heat (inflammation), tension and/or laxity
Relevant herbal actions: anti-inflammatory, circulatory stimulant, connective tissue lubricant, lymphatic, nerve trophorestorative, vulnerary

Herbal Allies

- Cinnamon essential oil
- Ginger
- Goldenrod leaf and flower
- Kelp
- Meadowsweet flower
- Peppermint essential oil
- Self-heal leaf and flower
- Solomon's seal root
- St. John's wort leaf and flower

The pain of an injured joint is your body speaking a warning to you. Heed it! Don't let a minor strain become a serious sprain. Rest the joint—but don't immobilize it; gentle movement allows blood to move through the injury site and speeds healing. Drink some bone broth (see Build-Up Broth), eat some seaweed, and work with herbs to reduce inflammation, improve blood exchange, and restore the connective tissues (tendons, ligaments, fascia).

One of the best methods for healing a sprain is alternating hot and cold compresses or baths. Heat exposure brings in fresh blood, while cold constricts the vessels and squeezes out stuck fluids. Alternate between 3 minutes of hot and 30 seconds of cold. Go back and forth a few times, and always finish with hot to bring fresh, healthy circulation to the area. See also Arthritis, and Joint Pain.

SOFT TISSUE INJURY LINIMENT

Makes about 8 fluid ounces (100+ applications, 30-day supply)

This is similar to Joint Liniment, but we add some extra vulneraries, lymphatics, and nerve-healing herbs to address the other types of tissue damaged in an injury.

3 fluid ounces ginger-infused oil

2 fluid ounces Solomon's seal-infused oil or tincture of
Solomon's seal

1 fluid ounce tincture of St. John's wort

1 fluid ounce tincture of self-heal

1 fluid ounce tincture of meadowsweet

40 drops peppermint essential oil

40 drops cinnamon essential oil

1. In a small bottle, combine the infused oils, tinctures, and essential oils. Cap the bottle and label it, including *Shake well before each use*.
2. Hold your palm over the bottle's mouth and tilt to deposit a small amount in your palm. Rub between your hands to warm the treatment, then apply to the painful joints.
3. Massage the oil into the joints until your hands no longer feel oily. Really work the liniment into the tissue.
4. Repeat the application 3 to 5 times per day. More is better!

JOINT SUPPORT DECOCTION

See here for the complete formula and instructions. Drink a quart or more of this decoction every day until the joint is well healed.

KELP WRAP

See here for the complete procedure. Prepare and apply a kelp wrap on the injured joint 1 to 3 times per day.

Stomach Ulcer/ Gastritis and *H. pylori* Overgrowth

Relevant tissue states: heat (inflammation), laxity (barrier compromise)

Relevant herbal actions: antimicrobial, astringent, demulcent, vulnerary

Herbal Allies

- Calendula flower
- Goldenrod leaf and flower
- Linden leaf and flower
- Licorice root
- Marshmallow
- Meadowsweet flower
- Plantain leaf
- Self-heal leaf and flower
- St. John's wort leaf and flower
- Yarrow leaf and flower

Inflammation of the stomach causes discomfort and interferes with digestion; when it gets severe, it can lead to ulcers. *Helicobacter pylori* is an opportunistic type of bacteria that proliferates when stomach acid is low. It's considered by conventional medicine to be "the" cause of many ulcers but is also a normal member of the gut flora for most healthy people, too. It only seems to cause problems when stomach acid gets too low, and eliminating it entirely with antibiotics is known to have some downsides. Still, when it does overgrow, it's necessary to get it back in check. At the same time, we can work directly to heal the ulcers and reduce inflammation—getting to the root of the problem and healing it there. See also Heartburn/Reflux/GERD.

COATING AND HEALING INFUSION

Makes 2 cups dried herb mix (enough for 12 to 16 quarts of tea)

If you have an active ulcer, this blend helps protect the sensitive tissue, coating the open wound. It also encourages healing of the underlying tissue. Sipping on this slowly throughout the course of the day gives the best results, as you'll be continuously bathing the ulcer with these soothing, healing herbs. Drink a quart or more every day.

¾ cup dried linden leaf and flower

½ cup dried marshmallow root

½ cup dried plantain leaf

¼ cup dried licorice root

1. In a small bowl, mix together all the herbs. Store in an airtight container.
2. Make a cold infusion: Measure 2 to 4 tablespoons of herbs per quart of water and place in a mason jar or French press. Pour in cold or room-temperature water and steep for 4 to 8 hours. (You can prepare this at night and have it ready for the next day.)

RESTORE ORDER INFUSION

Makes 2¼ cups dried herb mix (enough for 14 to 18 quarts of tea)

This combination of tissue healers and antimicrobials will corral *H. pylori* and other rambunctious microorganisms, while tightening and preventing further damage to the stomach lining. Drink a quart or more every day.

⅓ cup dried calendula flower

⅓ cup dried goldenrod leaf and flower

⅓ cup dried self-heal leaf and flower

¼ cup dried plantain leaf

¼ cup dried meadowsweet flower

¼ cup dried yarrow leaf and flower

¼ cup dried licorice root

¼ cup dried St. John's wort leaf and flower (see Tip)

1. In a small bowl, mix together all the herbs. Store in an airtight container.

2. Make a hot infusion: Prepare a kettle of boiling water. Measure 2 to 3 tablespoons of herbs per quart of water and place in a mason jar or French press. Pour in the boiling water, cover, and steep for 20 minutes or until cool enough to drink.

TIP: Omit the St. John's wort if you are concurrently taking pharmaceuticals.

Stress

Relevant tissue states: heat (agitation), tension

Relevant herbal actions: adaptogen, nervine, relaxant, sedative

Herbal Allies

- Ashwagandha root
- Betony leaf and flower
- Catnip leaf and flower
- Chamomile flower
- Elderflower
- Goldenrod leaf and flower
- Linden leaf and flower
- Rose
- Sage leaf
- St. John's wort leaf and flower

• Tulsi leaf

Everyone's stress is the same, and everyone's stress is different. We all have the same physiological response to stress—racing heart, shallow breathing, narrowed focus, heightened cortisol and blood sugar. But we react to potential stressors differently —something that bothers one person might roll right off another's back. Whatever is stressing you, herbs can help both as a short-term rescue in the immediate moment and in the long-term to build more "nerve reserve" and poise in the face of difficulties.

RESCUE ELIXIR

Makes 5 fluid ounces (40 to 80 doses)

When you need a quick respite from a hectic day, this is your best friend. This remedy works best if you can step away to a private space for a moment. Center yourself, breathe deeply for a few breaths, take your tincture, breathe a few more times, and return to the world. A little ritual goes a long way!

1 fluid ounce tincture of tulsi

1 fluid ounce tincture of betony

½ fluid ounce tincture of catnip

½ fluid ounce tincture of chamomile

½ fluid ounce tincture of elderflower

½ fluid ounce tincture of rose

¼ fluid ounce tincture of goldenrod

¼ fluid ounce tincture of sage

½ fluid ounce honey

1. In a small bottle, combine the tinctures and honey. Cap the bottle and label it.

2. Take 2 to 4 droppersful whenever needed.

EVERYTHING WILL BE FINE

Makes 3¾ cups dried herb mix (enough for 22 to 30 quarts of tea)

Another of our old reliables, this tea has gotten us and our clients through some tough times. It's great for those days when you feel like everything is falling down all around you—just make a cup, drink it as deliberately as you can, and let the warmth and relaxation move through you.

If your stress manifests with a feeling of heaviness and downtrodden exhaustion, include ¼ cup of dried goldenrod and/or sage. If it shows up as digestive upsets, include ¼ cup of dried chamomile and/or catnip. If your stress is chronic and ongoing, work consistently with Add Apt Aid, as well. Drink a quart or more every day.

1 cup dried betony leaf and flower

1 cup dried tulsi leaf

½ cup dried linden leaf and flower

½ cup dried rose petals

½ cup dried elderflower

¼ cup dried St. John's wort leaf and flower (see Tip)

1. In a medium bowl, mix together all the herbs. Store in an airtight container.
2. Make a hot infusion: Prepare a kettle of boiling water. Measure 2 to 3 tablespoons of herbs per quart of water and place in a mason jar or French press. Pour in the boiling water, cover, and steep for 20 minutes or until cool enough to drink.

TIP: Omit the St. John's wort if you are concurrently taking pharmaceuticals.

UTI

Relevant tissue states: heat (inflammation), laxity (barrier compromise)

Relevant herbal actions: anti-inflammatory, antiseptic, astringent, demulcent, diuretic

Herbal Allies

- Dandelion leaf
- Goldenrod leaf and flower
- Marshmallow
- Nettle leaf
- Thyme leaf
- Uva-ursi leaf
- Yarrow leaf and flower

You may have heard that urine and the urinary system are sterile. It turns out that's not true! Recent advances in analytical techniques have revealed that there is a large variety of microbes that live in the urinary system, both friendly and not so—just like in the intestines. So, a UTI, rather than simply being an "invasion" of pathogens, is actually a state in which unfriendly bacteria have been able to proliferate, and the mucous membranes of the urinary system have been compromised, losing their integrity and innate defenses. For this reason, herbal approaches to resolving UTIs are at least as focused on improving the health of the urinary mucosa as they are on killing microbes.

About cranberry juice: Drinking lots of liquids, any kind, helps eliminate or prevent a UTI by flushing out the troublesome bacteria. Cranberry juice is better than plain water, though, because it has some diuretic effects and makes it difficult for bacteria to adhere to the walls of the bladder and urethra. It's not usually enough to stop a full-blown infection, but if you start it early—when you first detect symptoms—and drink a lot (a quart or so a day), it will work! Choose unsweetened cranberry juice for best effects.

UTI TEA

Makes 2¼ cups dried herb mix (enough for 14 to 20 quarts of tea)

This blend calls on one of our most potent anti-UTI herbs: uva-ursi. For best results, drink this as soon as you're aware of your UTI—if you catch it on the first or second day, this is as close to a guaranteed win as you're going to find! Don't drink this for more than 2 weeks; uva-ursi is too strong for long-term use. If you're prone to chronic UTIs, convert this to a long-term-use formula for prevention purposes by simply removing the uva-ursi. (*If you have any preexisting kidney diseases, use this modified version only, even for short-term use.*)

½ cup dried nettle leaf

½ cup dried dandelion leaf

½ cup dried marshmallow leaf

¼ cup dried uva-ursi leaf

¼ cup dried goldenrod leaf and flower

¼ cup dried yarrow leaf and flower

1. In a small bowl, mix together all the herbs. Store in an airtight container.
2. Make a long infusion: Prepare a kettle of boiling water. Measure 2 to 3 tablespoons of herbs per quart of water and place in a mason jar or French press. Pour in the boiling water, cover tightly, and steep for 8 hours or overnight.

3. Drink a quart or more daily until symptoms resolve—and then one extra day after that. Also drink a quart of unsweetened cranberry juice, for good measure.

ANTISEPTIC SITZ BATH
Makes 1 sitz bath

Getting the herbs directly in contact with the affected tissues is always ideal. A sitz bath is an excellent remedy, and with this external application we can add apple cider vinegar to alter the pH of the urinary tissues—helping combat the infection.

½ cup dried goldenrod leaf and flower

¼ cup dried thyme leaf

¼ cup dried uva-ursi leaf

Boiling water, for infusing the herbs

¼ cup Epsom salts

¼ cup apple cider vinegar

1. In a quart-size jar, combine the herbs. Pour in enough boiling water to fill the jar, and cover it tightly. Let infuse for 20 minutes.
2. Strain the infusion into a dish basin or other container big enough to sit in.
3. Add the Epsom salts and vinegar. Stir to dissolve.
4. Add a bit more warm or hot water if necessary, so all your relevant parts are submerged when you sit in the soak. If you have cuts or abrasions, the vinegar may sting. In that case, dilute with water or more herbal infusion, or omit the vinegar. Soak for 15 to 20 minutes.
5. Repeat 1 to 3 times per day, depending on severity.

Wounds

Relevant tissue states: heat (inflammation)

Relevant herbal actions: antimicrobial, astringent, emollient, lymphatic, vulnerary

Herbal Allies

- Calendula flower
- Chamomile flower
- Goldenrod leaf and flower
- Kelp
- Marshmallow
- Pine
- Plantain leaf
- Rose
- Self-heal leaf and flower
- St. John's wort leaf and flower
- Yarrow leaf and flower

When working with a cut, scrape, abrasion, or other open wound, it's important to always follow the same order of operations:

Stop the bleeding. Direct application of pressure is usually the best way to accomplish this.

Clean the wound. Any particulate or foreign matter must be completely washed out of the wound or it will slow healing and allow infection to take root. A wound wash or soak with astringent, antimicrobial herbs is very effective for this stage.

Prevent or manage infection. Wound washes and soaks are also good here. Herb-infused honeys are extremely effective for this stage, serving both to disinfect and encourage healing. (Don't put tinctures directly into wounds unless you have no other option; even then, dilute them at 1 part tincture to 5 parts purified water, because alcohol inhibits cell growth.)

Encourage healing. Herb-infused honeys, poultices, compresses, and baths are all appropriate for open wounds. Once the wound closes (or if it was never very deep to begin with), you can transition to a salve. Choose herbs that are vulnerary, lymphatic (to drain blisters), and—especially in later stages—softening or emollient (to prevent scarring).

WOUND WASH

Makes 3 cups dried herb mix (enough for 10 to 20 quarts of wound wash)

If you're in a hurry, a simple wash with rose water or nonalcoholic witch hazel extract is very effective during the cleaning stage. After that, transition to soaks and compresses with a formula like this. In the later stages of wound healing, you may want to add ½ cup dried marshmallow or kelp for their emollient effects.

½ cup dried calendula flower
½ cup dried plantain leaf
½ cup dried rose petals
½ cup dried goldenrod leaf and flower
¼ cup dried chamomile flower
¼ cup dried self-heal leaf and flower
¼ cup dried St. John's wort leaf and flower
¼ cup dried yarrow leaf and flower
Salt, for the infusion

1. In a medium bowl, mix together all the herbs. Store in an airtight container.
2. Make a hot infusion: Prepare a kettle of boiling water. Measure 4 to 6 tablespoons of herbs per quart of water and

place in a mason jar or French press. Pour in the boiling water, cover, and steep for 20 minutes or until cool.

3. Stir in 1 teaspoon of salt for each quart of infusion you've made.

4. Soak the wounded part, or apply a compress over the affected area.

5. Repeat as frequently as you can, at least 3 times per day.

PINE RESIN SALVE

Makes 8 ounces (40-day supply)

Pine resin salve is our go-to for wounds that have closed or were never very deep. You can work with the resin of other conifers, too. Resin can be harvested directly from the trees— you'll find whitish globs of it along the trunk where branches were lost. Leave enough on the tree to keep the wound sealed —this resin is how the tree forms a scab! It will probably have bits of bark, dirt, insect parts, etc., stuck in it—don't worry! We'll filter that out during processing.

After gathering resin, use a bit of oil to wash your hands— soap and water won't work. Just drop a bit of any liquid oil you have handy into your hands and scrub as if it were soap. The resin will soften and separate from your skin. Then you can use soap and hot water to wash it away. You can use plain oil for infusing your resin, but starting with an herb-infused oil means you get the good actions of all these herbs, instead of just those the resin contributes.

6 to 8 ounces pine resin or another conifer resin

8 fluid ounces total calendula-infused oil, goldenrod-infused oil, and/or plantain-infused oil

1 ounce beeswax, chopped or grated, plus more as needed

1. In a small pan over low heat, combine the resin and infused oil and heat gently, stirring frequently. The resin will soften and dissolve, infusing the oil with its virtues.

2. Pour this warm oil through a few layers of cheesecloth. Wrap the mass that remains and squeeze it to extract as much oil as possible.

3. Prepare a salve using this resin-infused oil (see <u>here</u> for complete instructions).

4. Apply to the wound several times a day, using fresh, neat bandages each time.

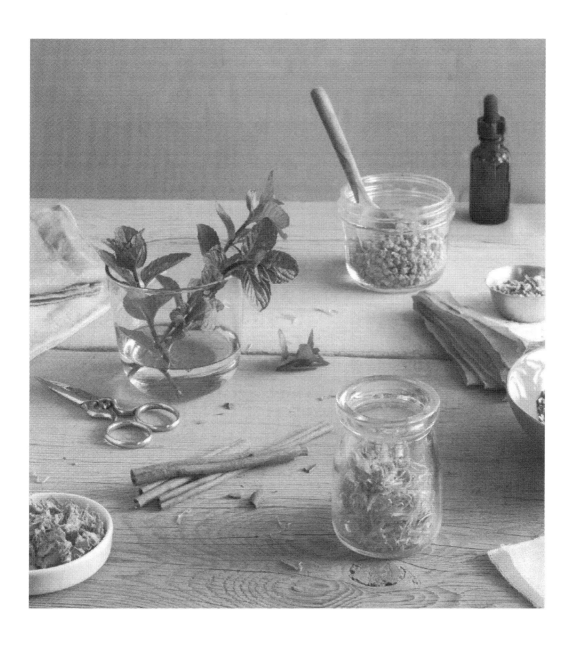

GLOSSARY

adaptogen: Normalizes endocrine function and increases the body's resilience in adapting to stress (for example: *ashwagandha, licorice, tulsi*).

alkaloid: A type of plant constituent, alkaloids often have strong effects on human physiology and are frequently the most potent chemicals found in an herb.

alterative: Supports nutrition, digestion, assimilation, circulation, or elimination and thereby improves the quality of the circulating fluids—blood, lymph, extracellular fluid (for example: *angelica, ashwagandha, calendula, dandelion, elder, garlic, milk thistle, nettle, St. John's wort*).

analgesic/anodyne: Relieves pain (for example: *ginger, goldenrod, linden, meadowsweet, mullein, St. John's wort, wild lettuce, yarrow*).

anticatarrhal: Tonifies mucous membranes in the sinuses and lungs; helps eliminate mucus (for example: *goldenrod, mullein, peppermint, pine, sage, thyme*).

antiemetic: Relieves nausea and prevents vomiting (for example: *fennel, ginger, peppermint*).

anti-inflammatory: Reduces inflammation through any of a wide array of mechanisms, e.g., antioxidant capacity, circulatory stimulation, relaxation, counter-irritation, etc. (for example: *garlic, ginger, goldenrod, linden, marshmallow,* *meadowsweet, milk thistle, mullein, peppermint, plantain, Solomon's seal, St. John's wort, thyme, yarrow*).

antilithic: Breaks up or prevents the formation of kidney or gallbladder stones (for example: *dandelion, goldenrod*).

antimicrobial: Inhibits the growth of or destroys bacteria, fungi, amoebas, and other microbial pathogens (for example: *angelica, calendula, chamomile, cinnamon, elecampane, garlic, pine, marshmallow, meadowsweet, mullein, peppermint, plantain, rose, sage, self-heal, thyme, tulsi, uva-ursi, wild lettuce, yarrow*).

antiseptic: Clears pathogens from infected tissue (for example: *goldenrod, pine*).

antispasmodic/relaxant: Prevents or relaxes muscle spasms, releases tension (for example: *ashwagandha, betony, catnip, chamomile, cinnamon, elderflower, fennel, ginger, goldenrod, mullein, peppermint, Solomon's seal, thyme, wild lettuce*).

antitussive: Quells coughing (for example: *elder, licorice, sage*).

antiviral: Helps the body fight viral infection (for example: *elderberry, self-heal, St. John's wort*)

anxiolytic: Reduces feelings of anxiety and promotes calm (for example: *betony, catnip, chamomile, linden, tulsi*).

aromatic: Pleasant-smelling herb that stimulates the gastrointestinal system, encourages circulation, and often stimulates or relaxes the brain and mind (for example:

angelica, catnip, chamomile, cinnamon, fennel, garlic, ginger, goldenrod, pine, linden, meadowsweet, peppermint, rose, sage, thyme, tulsi, yarrow).

astringent: Restores tone and causes constriction of tissues (for example: *betony, cinnamon, elderflower, goldenrod, meadowsweet, pine, plantain, rose, self-heal, Solomon's seal, uva-ursi, yarrow*).

biofilm: When certain bacteria and other microorganisms infect tissue, they can form a cooperative structure called a biofilm. This makes it more difficult for your immune system, antimicrobial herbs, and antibiotic drugs to fight the infection. Certain herbs, such as elecampane and uva-ursi, are proficient at disrupting biofilms.

bitter: Both a flavor and an action; stimulates digestive secretions, improving digestion and assimilation (for example: *angelica, dandelion root, elecampane, St. John's wort, wild lettuce, yarrow*).

carminative: Promotes digestion, expels gas, and relieves cramping in the gastrointestinal tract (for example: *angelica, catnip, chamomile, fennel, garlic, ginger, goldenrod, peppermint, sage, thyme*)

cholagogue: Promotes the flow and discharge of bile into the small intestine (for example: *dandelion root, fennel, peppermint*)

constituent: Any chemical naturally produced by an herb, particularly those that contribute to medicinal effects.

demulcent: Moistens, protects, and soothes mucous membranes throughout the body (for example: *cinnamon, kelp, licorice, linden, marshmallow, plantain, Solomon's seal*).

diaphoretic: Opens the skin channel of elimination, promoting perspiration and releasing heat (for example: *angelica, betony, calendula, elderflower, elecampane, ginger, linden, peppermint, sage, tulsi, yarrow*).

diffusive: Stimulates movement of blood from the body's center to the surface and periphery (for example: *angelica, betony, cinnamon, garlic, ginger, sage, tulsi, yarrow*).

diuretic: Increases the flow of urine (for example: *dandelion leaf, elder, fennel, goldenrod, pine, marshmallow, meadowsweet, nettle, self-heal, uva-ursi, yarrow*).

dysbiosis: A state of imbalance in the composition of the gut flora—too many unfriendly microbes, not enough probiotics.

emmenagogue: Promotes menstruation (for example: *angelica, elecampane, ginger, thyme, yarrow*).

emollient: Soothes and softens the skin (for example: *kelp, licorice, marshmallow, milk thistle, plantain*).

exhilarant: Lifts spirits and elevates mood (for example: *dandelion flower, rose, St. John's wort, tulsi*).

expectorant: Expels mucus from the lungs and throat; may be stimulating or relaxant (for example: *angelica, elecampane, licorice, marshmallow, milk thistle, mullein, pine, plantain, thyme*).

flavonoids: A large class of herbal constituents that often have anti-inflammatory or immune-stimulating effects.

galactagogue: Increases production of breast milk (for example: *fennel*).

grounding: Centers the mind in the body and settles restless thoughts (for example: *angelica, betony*).

hepatic: Strengthens and tones the liver (for example: *betony, catnip, garlic, milk thistle, plantain, sage, St. John's wort, tulsi, wild lettuce, yarrow*).

hepatoprotective: Restores healthy liver function (for example: *licorice, milk thistle, plantain*).

hypnotic: Induces sleep (for example: *wild lettuce*).

hypoglycemic: Lowers blood sugar levels (for example: *cinnamon, tulsi*).

hypotensive: Reduces elevated blood pressure (for example: *garlic, linden, Solomon's seal*).

immunomodulator: Elevates immune system activity if it is deficient, but reduces excessive activity, as occurs with autoimmunity (for example: *ashwagandha, self-heal, tulsi*).

inulin: A prebiotic fiber found in dandelion root, elecampane, and other herbs.

laxative: Promotes easy passage of stool (for example: *dandelion root*).

lymphatic: Stimulates the movement of lymph and disperses stagnation (for example: *calendula, self-heal*).

macerate: To soak herbal material in a menstruum (solvent) to extract its constituents into the liquid.

marc: Plant material that has been used in an extraction (tea, tincture, etc.) and has been separated from the menstruum (solvent).

menstruum: The liquid (alcohol for a tincture; water for tea) used to make an extract from an herb.

mucilage: A complex of long-chain polysaccharides that exudes from demulcent herbs when infused into cool water.

nervine: Calms nervous tension and nourishes the nerves (for example: *angelica, betony, catnip, chamomile, elecampane, linden, meadowsweet, rose, sage, St. John's wort, tulsi, wild lettuce*).

nutritive: Contains substantial amounts of vitamins, minerals, or phytonutrients (for example: *dandelion, elderberry, kelp, marshmallow, nettle, rose hips, Solomon's seal*).

phytonutrients: Any herbal constituent with nutritional or medicinal value, particularly those unique to herbs (i.e., bioflavonoids, terpenes, alkaloids, etc.).

prebiotic: Composed of starches and fibers that human digestive fluids don't break down, prebiotics are food for your friendly gut flora (probiotics).

pulse dosing: Taking herbs in smaller divided doses over the course of an hour, rather than a single large dose; a preferred strategy for remedies that improve sleep.

refrigerant: Directly cools the body, reducing fever and inflammatory excesses (for example: *rose, wild lettuce*).

resin: A blend of sticky constituents produced by some herbs or the sticky exudate of certain trees (e.g., pine).

rubefacient: Increases blood flow to the surface of the skin, dispersing inflammation and congestion in deeper areas (for example: *garlic, ginger*).

sedative: Depresses function or metabolic activity in an organ or tissue (for example: *catnip, chamomile, linden, mullein, wild lettuce*).

sialagogue: Stimulates the production of saliva (for example: *dandelion root, fennel, ginger, licorice, linden, marshmallow*).

stimulant: Increases activity or metabolism in a system, organ, or tissue, e.g., circulatory stimulant, immune stimulant (for example: *angelica, cinnamon, elderberry, elecampane, garlic, ginger, sage, yarrow*).

styptic: Arrests or reduces external bleeding due to astringent action on blood vessels (for example: *self-heal, yarrow*).

tonic/trophorestorative: Colloquial term for an herb that maintains or restores healthy function and increases vitality in a specific organ or type of tissue, e.g., cardiac tonic, nervous trophorestorative, etc., (for example: *chamomile, elecampane, kelp, mullein, nettle, Solomon's seal, St. John's wort*).

volatile: Herbal constituents are said to be volatile if they evaporate at room temperature or when exposed to boiling water. Essential oils are the distilled, volatile chemicals extracted from an herb.

vulnerary: Accelerates wound healing by promoting cell growth and repair (for example: *calendula, chamomile, goldenrod, kelp, marshmallow, meadowsweet, pine, plantain, rose, self-heal, Solomon's seal, St. John's wort*).

Final Words

I'm grateful to all the people who have helped and supported me along the way as I think back on the journey that inspired me to write this book. Writing is frequently a solitary activity, but to produce a work of this scope, a community is required. I am grateful to everyone who contributed to the creation of this book.

I want to thank my family first and foremost for their unwavering love and support. They are the reason I am the person I am today and the writer I am. Their belief in me has kept me going through the highs and lows of this project, and I am sincerely appreciative of their support.

Additionally, I would like to thank my friends, who have consistently provided me with motivation and support. I've been able to stay sane throughout the long days of research and writing thanks to your unwavering support, amusement, and encouragement. I appreciate the happiness you have brought into my life and the unwavering support you have given me as I have traveled this path.

I'd like to thank my peers and mentors for their advice and knowledge. I appreciate how generously you have given of your time and wisdom. Your willingness to share your expertise, perspectives, and resources has been priceless.

I would like to give a special thank you to everyone who helped with the research and writing of this book. I am appreciative of the insights you shared. Your interviews, criticism, and expertise have given my work more depth and nuance.

I want to express my gratitude to my editor and the publishing team for their unwavering assistance and knowledge. This book wouldn't exist without the suggestions, criticism, and encouragement you provided. I appreciate your commitment to and confidence in the worth of this project.

The institutions and groups that helped me with my research and writing deserve my gratitude as well. I am grateful to have had the chance to work with you because your resources, facilities, and knowledge have been so helpful.

I'd like to express my gratitude to the readers who will hold this book in their hands. This work was made for you, and I am honored to have the chance to share it with you. It is my sincere wish that it will enrich your life in some significant way and inspire, challenge, and amuse you.

I'd like to take this opportunity to express my gratitude once more to everyone who contributed to the publication of this book. Writing is a team effort, and we can only produce truly meaningful writing with the assistance and encouragement of others. I sincerely appreciate your help.

Abbyx .Z Austinx

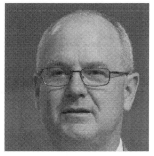

Made in United States
Troutdale, OR
05/15/2024

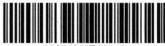

19874663R00210